CW01206721

# VISUAL TRAINING FOR TENNIS

Bill Patton

# Reviews

This book is a wow moment in tennis! The expertise brought forward with much of the latest research into the visual components of learning is cutting edge, culling information from multiple sports experiences. I wholeheartedly endorse the efforts to bring more education to this critical piece in learning the sport we all love. There will always be more to know on this topic, but this book has brought forward a large amount of digestible information to help you play, learn, enjoy and teach tennis better. A typically great Bill Patton offering!

**Dick Gould**
Emeritus: Men's Tennis Coach; Director of Tennis
17x NCAA Champion and Hall of Fame Coach
**Stanford University**
**Palo Alto, CA**


Bill Patton has written an insightful book on one of the critical factors for greater consistency: reading and reacting to the ball. Often ignored or overlooked by coaches, he also offers several highly practical exercises for improving this skill. I highly recommend it!

**Sean Brawley**
Player Development Coach
**The One Certified Inner Game of Tennis Coach**
Sean@SeanBrawley.com


The book did a great job articulating many of the things I felt, but didn't know how to verbalize clearly to students. Learning how to keep your eyes soft (Leonardo Da Vinci) till the last moment because they eyes can't hard focus for that long was great. It also helped explain the French system of training the eyes that I never really understood until reading about the dominant and non dominant eye. A great read for so many reasons!

**Michael Jessup**
Player Capital
Mountain View, CA


Bill Patton links the sports psychology concepts pertaining to anxiety with vision training. It's a great manual to understand this not often talked about subject. Most players are not fully aware of the untapped potential they can find when they learn visual skills. This is a great book!

**Carlos Llanes**
**TennisTiming and Focus**
Mundelein, IL

Bill Patton's book "Visual Train for Tennis" is a book every tennis player, tennis coach or teacher should read. In my humble opinion this is one of the best books to come out since "The Inner Game of Tennis" by Timothy Gallwey. I have been playing more than 60 years and teaching/coaching 46 of those years. I have read dozens of books on teaching and training tennis players. The content of this book is not only innovative, it truly makes you think and teaches us something uniquely new. The approaches offered into how we really see the ball and how we really do not see the ball, not to mention the court. We have so many teaching cliches' in tennis. This book will help you dispel some of the overused cliches', learning a better way, and help you understand how to teach visualization. This book is not only going to help me be a better teacher, it is already making me think about what I missed in my playing career and how I could have been a better player and will be a better teacher. Thank You Bill for "Opening our Eyes".

**Kenneth M Schuler**
USPTA Pro
Head Tennis Coach
Carondelet HS
Walnut Creek, CA


Tennis coaching that is much more than just focus and watch the ball!!! I've read many tennis coaching books and this one is very specific. If you are a coach or tennis enthusiast looking for drills and tips to implement in your game right now this book is a must read. There are golden nuggets that open your eyes literally to becoming a better tennis player one step at a time. Excellent and a quick read for visual training. Love how the chapters are chunked/bite size and to the point.

**Anonymous Amazon Customer**


Very valuable informations for every coach and instructor ... Must read!!!! We use the knowledge from this book to teach our advanced players the importance of the visual aspect in tennis. It is necessary to recognize this and to sensitize the players to it. Very well described and absolutely recommendable!!!!

**WGT Tennis**

Copyright © 2021 Bill Patton

All rights reserved.

ISBN: 1942597100
ISBN-13: 978-1-942597-10-0

Thank you:

**Styrling Strother** and **Brent Abel** for recognizing this as my best subject matter.

**Scott Ford** for your work, and time spent delving into this topic, and working with me directly on court.

**Sean Brawley** for the affirmation of being aligned with the 'Inner' way.

**Vic Borgogno** for suggesting much of the research material.

**Ken DeHart** for being an inspiration in terms of taking vision seriously.

**Lenny Schloss** with Billie Jean King's 'The Eye Coach for advancing the art of teaching.

**My Students** who put up with the mindset shifting in the lessons.

**My Wife Laurie** for allowing me sacred space to write with few distractions.

## *Table of Contents*

Chapter 1
**What Is Eye/Flow Coordination?**

Chapter 2
**Why Is 'Keep Your Eye On The Ball' And 'Watch The Ball' Are Not As Valuable As You Once Thought?**

Chapter 3
**Understanding The Interaction Between Anxiety And Perception To Advance To New Levels**

Chapter 4
**How To Move Past The Default Position Of "Overthinking"**

Chapter 5
**How To Get To Every Ball, Without Running Faster**

Chapter 6
**How To Reduce Errors, With Simple Ball Awareness**

Chapter 7
**Why You Might Not Be Aware That You Over Or Under React**

Chapter 8
**Why There Are Two Different Ways To Take In The Final Phase Of The Ball's Flight**

Chapter 9
**How To Reduce Visual Distractions Without Yelling 'Focus'**

Chapter 10
**Why I Don't Say "See The Ball, Through The Back Of The Strings"**

Chapter 11
**Why You Should Fine Tune Your Understanding Of Balance**

Chapter 12
**How Your Legs Help Your Eyes**

Chapter 13
**Why 'Hungry Eyes' Are Not The Solution, What To Do Instead**

**Chapter 14**
**How To Move Beyond Past Experiences
By Developing Visual Skills
For The Present And Future**

**Chapter 15**
**How To Effectively Model Strokes,
Learn Without Hitting A Ball**

**Chapter 16**
**Why You Can Ignore
Early Specialization Gurus**

**Chapter 17**
**How To Facilitate A Wide Variety Of
Visual Experiences On A Tennis Court**

**Chapter 18**
**Why Is Eye Dominance Fundamental Knowledge?
Using The Eye That Does Your Most Seeing**

**Chapter 19**
**What Are The Visual Considerations
For Each Shot?**

**Chapter 20**
**How Does The Time/Space Continuum Play Into Vision?
How Being Fully Present Improves Perception**

**Chapter 21**
**Why Is Ball Recognition An Evolving Problem?
Train And Care For Your Eyes**

**Chapter 22**
**Which Physical Exercises Strengthen My Eyes?
Take The Eye Muscle Workout**

**Chapter 23**
**What Do Visual Researchers Say Are Hidden
Capacities Of Vision? Reconciliation And Imagination**

**Chapter 24**
**When Do You Have A Lot Of Time To See The Ball?
How The Ball Slows Down For You, Or Not**

**Chapter 25**
**Why Are Sleep And Recovery A Fundamental?
How To Perform Closer To 100% More Often**

**Chapter 26**
**The Effects Of Environment
and Recovery On Visual Acuity**

### Chapter 27
**Which Factors Cloud Our Vision? How To Be Alert And Clear Minded On Court**

### Chapter 28
**Why Is Eye Protection Controversial? Use Different Methods To Protect Your Vision**

### Chapter 29
**What Are Coach's Opinions On Wearing Sunglasses?**

### Chapter 30
**How To Use Contact Point Awareness Exercises To Increase Efficiency**

### Chapter 31
**Can We Improve Our Focus? How To Improve Ability To Focus Without Saccads**

### Chapter 32
**Does Everyone Process Visually At The Same Speed? Understanding Factors That Effect Visual Processing**

### Chapter 33
**Why Move Away From Pinpoint Vision And Toward 'Bounce-Hit'?**

### Chapter 34
**Do We Have It Backwards? Challenge The Visual System With Overtraining, Before Introducing A Larger Ball**

### Chapter 35
**What Is The Sequence In Which We Check Visual Errors? Know The Five F's Of The Visual System**

### Chapter 36
**Stop Saying "Watch The Ball" And Learn To Give Full Attention To The Ball**

### Chapter 37
**On Court Visual Challenge Drills**

### Chapter 38
**How To Sharpen Objective Observations Of Your Shot Placements**

### Chapter 39
**What Are The Next Steps In Hitting More Targets Better?**

### Chapter 40
**Why Will The Visual And Kinesthetic Always Be Intertwined?**

### Chapter 41
**Why You Should Bring Your Ruler To The Court To Measure The Ball**

### Chapter 42
**Using Slow Motion Video to Support Visual Awareness**

### Chapter 43
**Is Anticipation Really Possible? How To Read And React Without The Guesswork**

### Chapter 44
**How To Prepare Your Eyes For Competition Without Sapping Your Energy**

### Chapter 45
**Is Being 'Always On' A Good Idea? How To Diminish Mental Visual Fatigue**

### Chapter 46
**Is It Really Possible To Be Perfectly Level Headed? How To Use Ideal Posture For Visual Acuity**

### Chapter 47
**Why Is It Important To Have An Origin Story?**

### Chapter 48
**How Bizarre Visual Events Can Create Empathy**

### Chapter 49
**What Should I Eat For Eye Health? Which Foods To Eat For Development, Improvement and Maintainence Of Vision**

### Chapter 50
**A Healthy Mind In A Healthy Body**

### Chapter 51
**Maintain Healthy Eyes - Early Warning Systems**

### Chapter 52
**How To Avoid Computer Vision Syndrome**

### Chapter 53
**Is There Social Proof Of These Principles? How Players Responded To Visual Issues, Learning To Win**

For every coach and player who is willing
to dig for the best information,
as though digging for precious metals

**How much better to get wisdom than gold,
to get insight rather than silver!
~ King Solomon**

## *Foreword*
## The Eyes Have "It"

I am an International Master Professional with the PTR, Master Professional with the USPTA and a High Performance Coach who has been teaching for....... a long time, let's say.

The one thing that changed my understanding of teaching sports, tennis specifically is how to use the eyes! It was always there before me, I had heard the familiar phrases most my life. But, one day there was an acute awareness, like an epiphany. I am sure it came as a result of my work with several people, Harvey Ratner, for sure Lenny Schloss and others that the eyes were what I was not seeing.

How to use the eyes correctly was the challenge. The eyes would tell me how fast, in what direction and how to adjust my feet to be in an optimal position to make or return a shot. The eyes would also tell me when and where I needed to direct my racquet to make contact with the ball. My eyes had also told me where my opponent was and what part of the court was open. All this seemed to occur without words from a coach. The coach would simply make me aware that this was possible, then get out of the way.

**The eyes connect with the brain in such a magical way to direct our body to perform a skill.**

Bill, in this particular book helps us to better understand the 5 "W's"; who would use this information, what is it all about, where it is used, when to use it and perhaps most importantly why use it to improve your athletic performance as a tennis player. I feel, no I know this is more effective and produces a more lasting result that most any technical tips I can give you to become a better player, coach and lover of this amazing game - tennis

**Ken DeHart**

408-892-3806
Director of Tennis - Silver Creek Valley CC
kendehart@aol.com
PTR International Master Professional
USPTA Master Professional
USA High Performance Coach
Author - Master Your Tennis Game

## *Introduction: What's New In The Fourth Edition*

Like a mechanic, who starts by checking the battery of a car that won't start, we want to start with the most obvious aspects of the system that is a tennis player.

**We start with the eyes.**

Taking a close and and multi-varied look at the visual system, which is not entirely complex when taken apart into segments, we then proceed one phase to the next, until a player has the best strategies for seeing the ball well throughout the entire point. Yes, there will be shifts in using different abilities and strategies. Shifts happen during the entire sequence, most of which occur on a subconscious level and are affected by a player's state of mind. This book draws in many sports psychology principles to aid in more clear, accurate vision.

The positive impacts on your game, how better vision of the ball leads to playing more on balance, hitting more cleanly, recovering more easily, reading and reacting to your opponent's shots. All of these things lead to you being more aware of their relative position, and a better ability to hit targets on the court, making you a better player, in many cases dramatically so. The most dramatic positive effect may be reducing mishits of the ball, outside of the sweet spot in the frame, and many other kinds of mistakes.

**Traditional teachings like, "Keep Your Eye On the Ball" and "Watch The Ball" are extremely limited or even damaging.**

Those players will find it hard to become a legitimate tennis player, or progress beyond the 4.5 level with limited visual skills. In fact, a large percentage of people who try tennis will quit the game, because they can't see the ball well enough. Another large group of players miss out on the joy of playing at their best possible levels, moving beyond the 4.0 level. With a few simple instructions on how to better use the mind/body connection, and they could be off to the races to 4.5 and beyond.

The obvious place to start in the mind/body connection is the physical aspect, the body. The eye is literally an extension of the brain. It is estimated that over 60% of the brain has some duties associated with vision input. Compared to the sense of touch (8%) and hearing (3%), the eyes are the by far the dominant input devices for your brain, and a conduit to your mind, wherever that is. This book is aimed as much of the mind/body connection between how your thoughts, modes of operation, and physical health affect your brain. The mind affects your eyes, but looking at that system in reverse, we start with what your eyes see, paying attention to good inputs, then reverse engineer, to make precisely measured responses.

The first chapter will immediately solve the most common and catastrophic error players make in their vision, that coaches make in their teaching, without the need for more gym time, or a crazy new diet. The first chapter alone, may be worth 10x the price of the book! When I teach a private lesson, those are usually the things I teach, and people go away amazed at how much better they played in one hour, even the 4.5 and 5.0 level players who train with me. However, **some players give up on improving**. Instead of ascending to new levels of competence and accomplishment in the game, they begin to plot their sandbagging, to win a USTA National Championship. Many coaches lack a full toolbox to help a wider variety of players, whom then they could retain as clients, club members, and simply tennis players, to grow the sport. You can instantly become a greater resource for the growth of tennis by improving your visual skills and those of people around you.

This work is evolving, and now in this fourth edition, there is more about how to win the mental warfare of a match, managing yourself in the best modes of brain operation, to allow your brain to work fast. You can also learn to force your opponent into a slow processing mode, giving you an edge in the point. You can control that, like a game of cat and mouse. If you have been trained to be like a cat, you have the advantage, but if you have not been trained that way, and the other player is a cat, then you are at a disadvantage. The best matchup will be between two cats! Watch how cats operate, they are very still with their eyes tracking an object before they pounce. The object moves first!

I am more and more convinced that visual skills are the #1 fundamental. The world's leading experts in visual ability for sports say that, if everyone is different, then the way they differ most is in their visual experience of the world around them. That is also true, in all ball sports. Every effort has been made to bring the cutting edge technologies and research to light, but only that which has social proof, in effectiveness for your game. There are some strange ideas that you might not understand immediately, and might not work for you, but they are understood and work perfectly for someone else. Not everything is for everyone. You should not come away from reading this, thinking that you have to do everything. In fact the opposite is true, find the ONE big idea and work that first.

Necessarily, there are some anecdotes and some science, one reviewer of the third edition, has said that the book is too much about me, but I don't think that's accurate. Telling a few stories of players and about my own struggles make it real, and every effort has been made to sprinkle those into the book without becoming overbearing. It is important to me to make this content accessible to the non-scientist, mostly because I don't like to read that stuff either. I went to great pains to share necessary science, and explain terms in full. If you have the third edition, this one is going to be well worth the upgrade.

The best thing you can do right now before continuing on with this book, is to **take some video of you playing**, so that you will have a 'before' set of images, then you can start to trace changes in your game, you can chart the amount of mishits you had, look for eye behavior, and also how quick your reactions are, then compare to video from practicing the principles in this work.

Bill Patton  4/25/2021

One

# What Is Eye/Flow Awareness?

*Every science consists in the coordination of facts; if the different observations were entirely isolated, there would be no science.*
*~ Auguste Comte*

## The Problem With Hand/Eye Coordination

There are major problems with this phrase, Hand-Eye Coordination. The most obvious of which, is that the eye comes first, not the hand. First, you must see the ball, then you can react, and the final piece is with your hand. What if we switch the words to Eye-Hand Coordination, that's fine but really footwork comes first, possibly three phases of vision occur, and finally the strings meet the ball, not the hand. Fascination with what the hand does, sabotages the natural flow of strokes.

I must have said over 50,000 times in my career, "more shoulders, less hands". This is because when you get in ideal position for the ball, you can create a great amount of flow of energy by engaging your core, rotating on the shot in non-linear stroke making. All of this is made possible by your eyes.

Now I also am taking the issue of coordination, because it presumes that the player has to perform some mental task. In reality your brain will do quite a lot of great coordination subconciously if you simply come to awareness of what you are doing. So, now the entirety of this book is going to be about different entry points to the systems of Eye-Flow Awareness. First you see the ball, then you align yourself with the ball for maximum efficiency of energy flow, and you will do that by simply learning to pay attention to the ball, discovering what gets in the way of this flow. When the vast majority of your shots are hit in flow, welcome to the zone.

**Eye-Flow Awareness is the name of the game.**

Two

## Why Is 'Keep Your Eye On The Ball' And 'Watch The Ball' Are Not As Valuable As You Once Thought?

*I don't know what 'genius' even means. It's just a matter of keeping your eye on the ball.*
~ Lindsey Buckingham

If you want to be one of the greatest living guitarists, and use 'keep your eye on the ball' as a euphemism for keeping your life mission in focus, fine! Just don't use that phrase on the sporting field, because it really makes no semantic sense at all, and there are so many more subtle skills that can be taught which will really help you. It's vitally important that the words we use to describe the experiences we are having are vital if we are going to convey it to someone else. There is no ball in guitar playing. This is not a knock on Lindsay, but it outlines a theme that runs through this book, that we can do a better job of describing things, and understanding them using the best thinking, which is sometimes expressed in words. Other times, it's hard to put into words the strategy that you use visually.

Recently, I heard a story of an amazing marksman who makes bullseye shots from miles away from the target, and he said that when he shoots, he 'has a hand in his mind that drops the bullet on the target'.

The physics of shooting a bullet from so far means that a calculation must be made for how much the bullet will be blown by wind, and how much it will fall because of gravity. Does that make sense to you? For me, I have to think on that a moment, let it sink in, then I think I understand. You can also think of similar strategies I have used in sports that require accuracy of ball placement.

### Conventional Wisdom v. More Accurate Information

One of the most common and least accurate pieces of advice given on a tennis court is 'keep your eye on the ball'. Ridiculous you say? Try this: make your eyes go from left to right back and forth, and pay attention to how clear, blurred, or choppy your vision is while you do that. As you can see, your eyes 'chatter' in their movement, when they try to follow something moving laterally.

So, why would we say something to ourselves or others, that could be misconstrued and done poorly? This easily leads to frustration for most people. Effective instruction must be something better than what has been taught for ages. The command to 'watch the ball' simply lacks any specificity. My pet theory on this is that those who heeded the instruction, succeeded due to inherent talent, or through sheer determination. Those exceptional ones, willed themselves to find a way to 'watch the ball' that worked for them, but they lacked the ability to express what they were doing. They then passed that apocryphal piece of advice along with the same poor level of instruction for the next generation to figure out on their own.

## Difficult Adaptations v. Easy Adjustments

Do you want to challenge your adaptability to the maximum, or would you rather shorten the learning curve, making an easy adjustment in how you see the ball? Would you prefer to go through periods of frustration, and stagnation, or amaze people when they ask you how long have you been playing, and it's only been a few weeks or months? When last season you were a 3.5 and you now are a strong 4.0, people will wonder what happened. Learning awesome visual skills can take your game up a whole notch in a short while. Unfortunately, too many people are relying on their adaptability to solve visual problems, and they might go months or years before they discover a strategy. 50% of adult tennis players who take up the game do not continue playing, and it's my contention that a large percentage of them quit because they don't see the ball well. The symptom that is always discussed is that they couldn't find someone to play, but a large percentage of those people were not good enough for someone to want to play.

## Learning Visual Skills First

We can be much more efficient, saving a lot of time and effort by teaching specific skills for different parts of the ball's travel. We can shorten the learning curve with all players and especially new ones with player specific skills to build what they need to improve and they should be taught first, now, ahead of any stroking techniques. Instead, up until now we have continued to give the same sort of non specific instruction repeated over and over to ourselves and others. The general lesson here for you and coaches, who want to help themselves and others, is to put a finer point on helping players discover how exactly it works for them. We want to use language that accurately describes what is actually happening. As with everything, we have discovered that no two people see exactly the same way. A coach the other day expressed, that he found out his player was nearly blind in their non-dominant eye, that revealed quite a bit about why the student struggled with certain objectives on court.

## A Multitude Of Visual Influences

Vision plays a role in every shot, so be sure to examine how you are seeing the ball, or not, at any given time, starting with the beginning of the sequence when the ball comes out of the opponent's frame. There are times that it's best for you NOT to see the ball for a moment, the moment immediately after you have made contact, where following through and recovering on balance are more important than seeing the ball. Players try to see the ball so hard at all times, that they compromise their finish, and find it hard to recover for the next ball. Then we can begin to look for breakdowns in the visual system at times when we need to see the ball beginning with the forward phase of the opponent's swing, to pick up something called Kinematics - more on that later.

Like a mechanic, who starts by checking the battery of a car that wont start, we want to start with the most obvious thing that occurs first to develop the visual system. We then proceed on to the next phase and the next, until a player has the best strategies for seeing the ball well throughout the entire point, and there will be shifts in using different abilities and strategies that happen during the entire sequence. The positive impacts on your game of playing more on balance, hitting more cleanly, recovering more easily, reading and reacting to your opponent's shots, being more aware of their relative position, and a better ability to hit targets on the court, all these things are going to make you a better player.  Especially in the case of reducing mishits of the ball, outside of the sweet spot in the frame.

Three

# Understanding The Interaction Between Anxiety And Perception To Advance To New Levels

*Tennis is a game of emergencies* ~ Peter Burwash

When we look out on the world, or the tennis court, what do we see? Our perception, our understanding of what might happen, is colored by our relative anxiety or calm, our confidence or lack of confidence. We discussed earlier that heightened anxiety can create a higher rate of blinking, but anxiety can have even more devastating effects on perception. In the realm of education, the concept of the *affective filter* is an important one. Essentially, this means that our anxiety has an affect on what we are able to see, process and places a limit on what we can learn. When we experience high anxiety, little in the way of learning happens. It can be quite difficult to deal with a fast moving, spinning, bouncing ball, especially when coming from a place of inner turmoil. We would do very well to create low anxiety learning atmospheres for ourselves and others. Reflect on times that you were very anxious about something, and how difficult it was to take in new information, or maybe you are running late, now it's extremely difficult to see your car keys, even though they are sitting out in the open. When we have plenty of time and are not in any rush at all, it's generally easy to see what we need to do.

## Trait and State Anxiety

Everyone comes from a slightly different place on the anxiety spectrum. Rainer Martens did a landmark Sport Psychology study in the 1970s, where he split out the somatic, or physical effects, and experiences of anxiety from the mental experience, known as cognitive anxiety. As it turns out, when you are less anxious mentally, there is a strong correlation to better performance. In measuring people's responses, he found large populations of people with widely varying levels of anxiety from very high to very low.

**What Dr. Martens discovered was that as mental anxiety diminishes, and physical anxiety reaches a mid point, then you most likely have the best recipe for success.**

So, very high anxiety people will need to slow down, calm down, but low anxiety people might actually need to activate their physical anxiety to raise it up to the midpoint. The story of Bill Russell, one of the great champions in the history of basketball vomiting before every game is a pretty extreme example. The interesting thing about his case, is that he seems to be one of the most relaxed people you might ever want to meet, off the basketball court. My pet theory, I have put into practice with my relaxed players is to first raise the intensity of the situation, before managing to bring the anxiety level into the appropriate zone. I have had other, higher anxiety players who need to do some serious breathing, managing their thoughts before they go on court, and others who are just always ready to play, needing no interventions, while others need to raise their heart-rate and get themselves pumped up.

All of these interventions are there to help get your body and mind managed into an ideal performance state. There is no one cookie cutter approach. When I was younger, I tended to have more anxiety, so I created some rituals that included deep breathing and visualizing before my match. I would also avoid getting into conversations within 30 minutes of my match time, to allow me to clear my head and get everything directed at my match. If you are too anxious, you are not going to be able to see as clearly, and if you lack intensity, then you won't have the right amount of alertness. Reducing your mental anxiety, and bringing physical tension, alertness and reaction to a mid point is ideal.

## Anxiety, Patterns and Perception

To the beginning player every ball is an emergency. As you move along in your game, fewer and fewer balls fall into that category. It's only natural that perceiving something as an emergency is going to have an effect on the amount of nervousness you feel, giving you something for which to worry. Many players, who might normally be fairly low anxiety, because of they way they have been trained, have a medium to high level of anxiety as they play. Our society teaches us to place more value on the competition and it's outcomes than we should, thus raising the stakes and the pressure people feel as they play. They worry about not doing it right, missing something, disappointing people, etc.

**Even top players can experience the ball as something that causes great anxiety.**

The eminently quotable Andy Roddick said, "Coming to the net against Nadal is like running head first into oncoming freeway traffic." Players who begin to gain confidence might rally well, but when a ball comes appreciably faster, to their backhand or high in the air, may experience much higher anxiety levels on those particular shots. When you have a particular shot that that they are less comfortable with, then the amount of fear can escalate based on the challenge level. In this way, your past experience of failures, can affect the accuracy of your vision of the ball, especially if you replay those mental programs as you prepare for the shot. Creating strong visual cues, and using very strong timing techniques can greatly reduce the amount of anxiety that players experience for any shot, building new more confident habits to gradually replace the old ones.

## Regress, Build Confidence, Progress

You must get into the business of developing basic confidence in a particularly challenging shot for you, with simple strategy, while increasingly developing mastery at different levels. Increasing competence, increases confidence, and vision of the ball will improve with it, vision of the ball will then increase competence because of the reduction in anxiety. Then you don't freak out because 'Oh no! A high topspin to my backhand!', because you have trained in how to deal with that shot.

As was stated earlier, the experience of vision is mainly made up of subconscious decision making, from within our brains, made up of processing our past experiences of the ball. Perhaps, it is the lack of experience in dealing with many different kinds of tennis shots, that makes the brain work overtime to react to what seems like an emergency. When I teach beginners, and they begin to have rally skills, then we go about the business of recognizing a short low ball, and a high bouncing deep ball, because both of those require specific skills.

## It all starts with immediate recognition.

Ball recognition was a teaching fad in the tennis professional circles about 10 years ago, but I'm not hearing about it much anymore, and this visual training content is attempting to replace the hodgepodge of information, with something that attempts to be complete. When you don't recognize what kind of shot is coming, it fools you, making it more difficult to time, or even react to it's initial flight, then you are in trouble. The incredibly well trained player in shot recognition is not easily fooled, even by those who have incredible ability to disguise their shots.

## Finding New Challenge Levels

As we improve, fewer and fewer shots invoke the same type of anxiety, but conquering the fear of a faster, higher, or different kind of shot is a major factor in moving up the levels. The ability then to make better decisions and shot selections, as the game starts to look more like ping pong, is where new levels of the game can be found. We may then bump into the upper levels of comfort zone in terms of how good do we believe we can be. Players at the upper level of their comfort zone can still rely on their reflex of seeing and doing without overthinking, seemingly automatically responding in the best possible way. Once we are out of our comfort zone, then our technique may fall apart momentarily.

## Higher Levels, Greater Anxiety

Even when a player improves their skill level, their self image may cause them to play at a lower level, because they don't yet believe they are as good as today's performance. Visualization can be helpful in those cases for players to begin to see themselves as better, deserving to be on a higher level. Players with low self esteem may become lazy, not using all the tools at their disposal.

**The mental and emotional aspect of attentional control is something to be aware of, and may need to be addressed in some players.**

My advice is to pay close attention, to see if performance and ability to see the ball slips back down to a lower level, then ask the player questions about how they perceive the own ability. If the eyes are the window of the soul, then when the soul has unresolved issues in the outlook for success, vision can be clouded. The connection between our self concept, our anxiety levels and our vision is hard to pin down exactly, but we can have a discussion and work to discover root causes, realizing that when one improves, the other two necessarily will need to improve as well.

Four

# How To Move Past The Default Position Of "Overthinking"

*Therefore, you, knowing I am not a fool,
would clearly not place the poison in front of yourself.
~ Vicini (in The Princess Bride)*

It's a fairly deeply ingrained part of human nature to want to get feedback on how we are doing. However, the default position for adults seems to be overthinking everything, and that gets them inside their head, and not looking through their eyes very well. It's very common that tennis players will want to know the outcome of their shot, judging it as good or bad as soon as they hit it.

Many players go through their entire tennis careers hitting the ball, turning their head while they are hitting it, to judge how was it, and then instantly try to diagnose what they did well or wrong.

This follows a medical model. In medicine, the doctor examines the patient, tries to determine what is wrong, then prescribes medicine, physical therapy or some other path to wellness. They are always looking for something wrong. In the ideal coaching model, the coach assumes that the player can become the expert, assisting them through guided discovery, to help them find their way.

## Leave Your Mind, Come To Your Senses

In the visual training for tennis coaching model, a player leaves their mind, coming to their senses. Which does not mean that a player should not think, but the typical thinking players do on court is maladaptive. Players often are in constant self evaluation mode, which takes away from simple awareness of what they are doing. Having a checklist of objectives like: turn your shoulders, prepare racquet, backswing, contact, follow-through and then finish, are simply happening too fast for a player to manage, but they use up a huge amount of their brain's CPU power which takes away from ability to see the ball. They also, then use subjective judgements about their shots, saying good shot, bad shot, pretty good, pretty bad and a lot of confused shades of subconcious not knowing how to label, which leads to worry, doubt, tension, frustration and even pretty deep and dark self talk.

As Tim Gallwey states in Inner Game of Tennis, players can go from a mishit forehand, to I am a bad player, to I am a bad person, in their minds quite easily.

Then the player turns their attention outward for solutions, and the coach is expected to engage with their illness, administering the answers to the murky questions that plague them. Still other players come to tennis as though it were a performance art, and that the point is to look good while doing it, and those produce flowery movements that reflect what they think they see from professional players, resulting in forearms that rotate this way and that, follow throughs below the belt, and many other strange and dangerous moves that are their attempt to mimic the top players.

### Triggers, Impulses, and Responses

It's far better for you to instead leave all of that, learning to calmly, see clearly what you are doing, and tuning into the feeling of your shot when you really like the outcome, and pretty much dismissing most other attempts. Looking for patterns is also a good objective, because when you notice a certain tendency to a certain maladaptive

### Habits

People are generally so fascinated with seeing the outcome of there shot, judging it good or bad, analyzing what went well or wrong, and strategizing how to do better, that they compromise their simple vision and trusting their eyes and brain to work together like they do every single day.

### Intuition

People intuitively, or because of former training tend to do certain things that actually don't work very well. They try to line things up in straight lines, even when an angled a approach works better, and they also intuitively will attempt to keep pinpoint vision of the ball, which only leads to difficulties in other areas, rather than using the eyes in the way they best work. Of course, moving forward we are going to walk through many different ideas, skills and drills that will give you new insights and things to practice.

### Preconceived Notions

Watching tennis on TV can be a bit deceiving, because what you are seeing is a two dimensional image, but then will need to translate that into 3D action. The camera angles from the back, make it difficult, because you can't easily see how short or long the players backswings or follow throughs are, so there is some unintentional deception to learning visually on a screen. YouTube and other platforms that offer side views and slow motion video is a far superior way to consume learning about strokes. The caution there is that you don't become The Frankentstein's Monster of tennis. Mimicking your favorite pro is fine, but not necessarily their idiosyncratic motions, you might find your own, so even when learning visually, be sure to learn how you do that. Play like yourself.

Five

# How To Get To Every Ball, Without Running Faster

*It's attention to detail that makes the difference
between average and stunning.
~ Francis Atterbury*

Once you know how to hit the ball at all, everything else on a tennis court is about saving time and space, and/or taking them from your opponent. How would you like to get every ball without having to run faster? How would you like to get more balls at a smooth, under control pace? Would you like more time to get into the most efficient possible position to hit great shots? Do you want to decrease your errors and increase the errors your force in your opponent? Sounds too good to be true? It's not. First you have to admit that there is something that you are not quite doing right on the tennis court.

**Almost 100% of the players I meet for the first time think they are seeing the ball out of the opponent's racquet, but their definition is off by a little or a lot.**

It's off by a little when they still pick up the ball fairly early in it's flight, and those are usually the 4.0/4.5 players. The players really struggling are the ones who only give a casual glance, then they are the ones for whom the ball seems like a surprise. It's like your asking yourself how the ball got there so quickly, or you have an 'uh oh' moment, because all of a sudden it's way over there, or it's a mishit ball that barely cleared the net. The problem of slow reactions, poor ball recognition, and being ill prepared to play the strategy you want to play is one of seeing the ball too late.

### See The Ball At The Best Time And Place

You can see the ball on time, or late coming toward you, there is no early. The word anticipation is not a great one, because there is an element of guessing that happens, and when you guess wrong, then you find yourself out of position. Yes, of course, there are a handful of times on a tennis court where you are so far out of position that you have to guess, or you can sprint to the open court, simply to try to get your opponent to change their shot. These are the exceptions to the rule, they are not the strategy of how to see the ball better and respond to it more quickly in a general sense.

## Your Mindset Should Be One of Reading and Reacting

You may be a person who does not have the fastest reactions to visual stimuli, and we are all different, but even if you have lightning fast reflexes and can see quickly, you most likely will need to train your first response. I have yet to meet a player on court who did not need to train their response to the ball. Sometimes I use 'molasses in January' to describe their movement, a thick liquid in a cold environment does not move like mercury.

## Finite Reaction Time

There is a finite amount of reaction time that simply is not conquerable. Minimum it takes .04 of a second for the impulse of seeing an object to trigger the ability to respond. For some it's longer, and I don't want to go down the rabbit hole about whether that can be trained, but suffice it to say that if you are 100% healthy, eating right, fit and have good or well adjusted vision, then you have probably maxed out your ability to have the fastest possible finite reaction time. However, the trained decision making response time is what most people don't realize that they have much more control over in how they play. You can urge yourself on to do better in this regard.

## Practicing Fast Reactions

Great coaches and players have been subjected to an almost 'Simon says' approach to making the first move. The coach will hold a ball up in the air, and when they move it from one side to the other, then players have to quickly prepare and maybe even take a first step in that direction. In practice, you might find that you have to push yourself to make your first move immediately after seeing the ball.

## When And Where: Opponent's Contact Point

So now, finally, what to do? Use scanning skills, because people try to focus too much, and we will get into that more later. Scan to the other side of the net, so that you can take in the whole player in your eyes, while giving your attention to the ball coming out of their frame. When you see the ball going into and out of their frame, while also seeing their relative body position, your brain takes in many tiny cues, and you see better read what kind of shot is coming.

**Vic Braden, the face of sports science in tennis for many years, shared that once the ball is out of the frame of the opponent by 2, that your brain with 95% accuracy knows where it's going.**

So that means that within a few feet, you know where to run. Watch professionals and see how quickly they respond to the ball out of the opponent's racquet. See the ball out of the frame, every time, and push yourself to have the quickest possible reactions and you can save a lot of time and space on every shot, and take advantage of many more opportunities to take away time and space from your opponents.  As you continue up the ranks, as the ball speeds and spins up more and more, then you will need to advance your ball recognition, reaction and first step skills.  It gets a lot more fun when you do.

Six

# How To Reduce Errors, With Simple Ball Awareness

*You have to know what you are doing.*
*~ Torben Ulrich*

Failing to give full attention to the ball coming out of the strings of the opponent, is the most universally damaging issue in most player's game. A breakdown in fully attending to that moment in time and space will mean missing out on vital information about the incoming shot. That explains how you get fooled by the shot, when it seems to arrive faster than you thought, you find your self slow to move, you get jammed by the ball or do a lot of reaching. However, when you use scanning skills to the opponent, after you have completed your shot to simply find the ball out of their strings, your brain gathers massive data, and helps bypass your thinking mind to get you moving right away to the ball, and then depending on how well you track the ball, then you will find an amazing improvement in the efficiency and accuracy of your movement.

## Train Lightning Fast Preparation

The next step would be to train yourself to turn and move as quickly as you can read what is coming out of the racquet. I challenge my players to make their first move to the ball by the time the ball is out two feet, they don't argue with me, and I also know that it might be an impossible standard, but the better they get at it, the more they improve as a player. You can move on time with the ball, or late, there is no early, in fact when you move early, that's when a good opponent will hit behind you.

## Look Big, See Small

To be clear, what you can do is take a bigger view of the other side of the court, look at your opponent or practice partner, but locate the ball coming out, as your brain will also start to pick up on cues from your opponent. You will be better able to detect when the opponent has mishit, when they are off balance, when they are moving forward to take the ball on the rise, or especially when your shot has put them in trouble and you can move in to take some space away, or prepare for a weak reply.

## What Is Scanning?

Scanning is what you use when you are in a clearing of a forest and you hear a noise, and your eyes take a larger view to find some type of movement in the trees to locate what kind of animal it might be, or even what else might have caused the noise. In the same way, but in a smaller field of vision you will detect the level and kind of threat caused by the ball the other player hits. Finding where it's going is far more powerful, and helps the data cross your brain in the fastest pathway for success. If you are thinking what kind of shot it is, how do I hit it back, or making a decision about when should you move, then you those thoughts go through the 'thinking' brain and you will be hundredths of a second slower, and thus at a disadvantage to the player who uses their unthinking brain to simply go to where the ball is going without unwanted delays. As we move along in this book we will use more and more refined skills to help you dial in your very best contact.

## Overestimating Scanning Performance

Most players when asked if they are seeing the ball out of the opponent's frame will tacitly say yes, that they are doing it. When really pressed to pay complete attention, to be fully present with the moment, they realize that they are not. My friend Styrling Strother, and author and coach asked his son if he sees the ball coming out the racquet, and of course he said yes. They then went on court to test it out. Pierce, the rising 13 year old said that, 'When I really started to see the ball come out, it was like I felt like I always knew where you were going to hit!', and his game took an amazing spike upward. It's interesting how low our standards are when it comes to this vital aspect, and that it can be actually a fairly difficult training exercise to see the ball coming out of the frame close to 100% of the time.

## Accept The Challenge

I'm guessing that reading, you probably think that you always see the ball coming out of the strings, but then next time you go out on court, give all your attention to the ball immediately at the time your opponent strikes it. One thing that's curious to me, is that when my players begin to do this in their first lesson with me, they make a quantum improvement instantly, but when I ask them if they were reacting better to the ball, they often say no, even though to my eyes the answer is obviously yes. As a player you might notice a huge difference, or you might have to trust a subtle difference. If you have some recent video of you playing, make new video of you practicing this, and then compare to the old video. It can be hard to see a subtle difference in the effect, but as a coach you can video tape your player before, then give them the advice to see the ball out of the frame. Then take the after and compare, so that the player can see the effect from outside of their normal experience.

Seven

# Why You Might Not Be Aware That You Over Or Under React

*There is a moment between stimulus and response.*
*~ Victor Frankl*

In 1970, Rainer Martens did a series of landmark studies, where he discovered two very important assertions. The first is that your mental anxiety is not necessarily connected to your physical feelings of anxiety. To get technical for a moment, your mental anxiety is also known as Cognitive Anxiety (CA), and the physical is called Somatic Anxiety (SA). In general he found that when Cognitive Anxiety is lower, or Confidence is Higher, players perform better. When players are at a midpoint of Somatic Anxiety, then that generally gives a better performance. If you aren't too tight, but also aren't too loose. Anxiety also has an effect on your visual performance.

## Cognitive Anxiety - Confidence v. Worry

When your, CA is high, you are likely to be worried or overthinking your performance, and that takes away precious brain activity away from your visual performance. When your CA is low, and confidence is high, then you have all your mental faculties available to see what's happening. If you are wondering about over-confidence, yes, it can happen, but it's actually pretty rare in research settings. There are two times I see overconfidence, when a young player starts to have their first major success, because of a lack of maturity, they often become overconfident immediately, followed by an experience a big let down, created by their new expectations.

Another time is when an already confident person is surrounded by confident people, they may respond by creating a much more difficult scenario for themselves to escape. They paint themselves into a corner in words or deeds. In the vast majority of people, a lack of confidence is the true issue, and it sometimes can lead to 'acting out,' pretending to be more confident than you are. Not all data reflects the real truth of what is happening, so even those that report feeling extremely confident, might not be telling exactly how they are really feeling.

## Somatic Anxiety - Peak Taut State v. Tight or Loose

When your SA is at a midpoint, then you have the alertness to find the ball, move to it and track it. If you are excessively nervous, this can lead to tightness that may slow you down, make your vision a bit more erratic, and have you overreacting to shots. Most beginners, not knowing that tennis is actually an easy game, come to it with a mentality of always trying hard, and then they miss easy shots, directly because their mind set caused them to be more anxious. Of course, there are those who are a bit more casual about most things, and they don't bring enough effort. Those with low SA will be likely to not be fully alert to the ball. They might not make a quick first move to the ball. They might also stop early to reach for it, instead of continuing all the way to an ideal position to strike it. They may have more of a 'good enough' attitude about playing. They need to raise their intensity a notch or two to succeed. The issue here is alertness and attention. In a later chapter we are going to discuss 'hungry eyes', which is something I see in the 3.0/3.5 crowd quite often.

## Trait v. State Anxiety

The second major discovery by Martens was, the difference in a performance setting between Trait and State anxiety. Trait means how you generally are, which is also trainable, but more gradually over time. I myself used to have high trait anxiety, but using the principles in this book, have learned to slow myself way down, and people describe me as 'Zen,' when really I prefer to be acknowledged for knowing how the brain works, and that Zen fits nicely into the brain science. Some people are simply wired to be more anxious than others, and some folks have had experiences that influence their anxiety that others have not had. An example would be those who don't realize the true danger of a situation, and those who do and how surprising the reaction is when those that know the danger, try to explain to those who don't. So you might be high, medium or low anxiety. If you want to take Marten's test, go to the Human Kinetics website and find his works on Competitive Anxiety in the early 1970s.

Your State Anxiety is how anxious do you feel right now. This can be manageable. It might take more work for those who have extremely low or extremely high Trait Anxiety. An example is Bill Russell, who is a very low trait anxiety individual, such a cool customer, but he would get himself extremely worked up before a game, and the legend has it that he would vomit before every game. From that heightened point of driving himself high into anxiety, he then would come down into a performance state. No one basketball person has ever down with Russel did, winning an NCAA Championship, an NBA championship as a player, and a coach. His Boston Celtics teams were one of the most dominant dynasties in all of sports. His behavior is rare.

In general low trait anxiety players are more likely to need to pump themselves up some physically, and more high trait anxiety players may need to bring themselves down both mentally and physically.

Also, keep in mind, that feeling a bit nervous is a great thing, because it means that your body is producing adrenaline, which you need to have the energy to perform. How you modulate that with your breathing, thinking, and scanning your body for the ideal balance of tension and relaxation can take some years of practice to perfect.

## Reactions

All of this is to explain the factors that play into how you will react to the ball. In general, higher anxiety states will create over reactions, conversely, too low of Somatic Anxiety can lead to an under reaction to the ball. Most commonly, people are too anxious and they make mistakes, but while less common, some people need to urge themselves to bring a bit more intensity to the situation. This is a major point for my on court coaching with teams. "Maintain Your Intensity," which my players know means that if they are too intense, they need to breathe and shake out some tension. If they are not intense enough, they might need to do a little dance on court to get their heart-rate up.

**There seems to be a pretty strong correlation between heart-rate and intensity.**

Of course, when play gets very intense, then you need the full time between points, and good deep breaths to bring heart-rate down. Another pro tip is that research shows that players serve better when their heart-rate is lower, and they return serve better when it's higher. An intense baseline rally often gets your heart-rate into the 160-180 beats a minute range. An intense point at the net can create a response in the 180-200 beats a minute which means very close to, or at a player's maximum heart rate. So, you might have to get up or down, but during a match you will need to manage your intensity point to point for a better visual performance of alertness, and low anxiety. If you are winning a lot of points easily, it's highly likely you will need to avert a dip in intensity, and if you are in a very tough match, then point to point you will need The 16 Second Cure. Every match has it's intensity challenge that will affect how well you see the ball.

## Discovery

The topic of how you identify your anxiety and how it differs from others, then digging into solutions that work best is worth the effort. I want to challenge you right now, that perhaps you have settled for a good answer that gives you moderate success, but if you keep digging, you likely can find better ones that lead to greater achievements. I have met so many players who seem to have a strategy for having clarity, but then when we dwell a while on the issue, it doesn't take long for an overreaction, overthinking, or the opposites to occur. We then set about finding what will work for them. Many of those answers are above, and even more solutions are found in future chapters. The answer might

NOT be to do it like Djoker, Fed or Serena.

Eight

# Why There Are Two Different Ways
# To Take In The Final Phase
# Of The Ball's Flight

> I don't like ass kissers, flag wavers or team players.
> I like people who buck the system. Individualists. I
> often warn people: Somewhere along the way,
> someone is going to tell you, there is no "I" in
> team.' What you should tell them is, 'Maybe not.
> But there is an "I" in independence, individuality
> and integrity.' Avoid teams at all cost. Keep your
> circle small. Never join a group that has a name.
> If they say, "We're the So-and-Sos," take a walk.
> And if, somehow, you must join, if it's unavoidable,
> such as a union or a trade association, go ahead
> and join. But don't participate; it will be your death.
> And if they tell you you're not a team player,
> congratulate them on being observant."
> ~ George Carlin

People are huge fans of other great players, mimicking as much of their games as they can. When it comes to Federer in particular, he has been held up as the paragon of virtue, perfection when it comes to seeing the ball well, and having ideal strokes.

Many times, I have shared about seeing a tennis magazine that put a green circle on the picture of Federer, as he focuses on the ball, all the way into his strings.

He allows his head to direct his eyes at contact until he needs to move. In that pictorial analysis, another professional player will then be used for comparison, and the author places a red X on their picture, meaning that it's bad, or at the very least it's not as good as Fed. Do you find it strange that the person pictured is a grand slam championship winner? How many of us would love to be a one time winner of a Grand Slam tournament? Can their visual strategy be all that bad?  The champion pictured looks slightly ahead of the contact point, like Serena Williams, or Andre Agassi do, obviously two of the greatest champions in the history of tennis.  Approximately half of the tennis players in the world will do themselves a disservice by trying to emulate Federer in this instance, and the other half will do themselves a favor. It's important to know which one you are.

## Social Proof

While I don't have a study to point to, that shows approximately 50% of players have one style of seeing the final phase of the balls flight, and the other half another style, I do have my own social proof in which I am very confident. I have tested my own players, but to confirm that these things are not subject to bias, or that only people in my area experience this, I have tested players in Phoenix, Atlanta and Birmingham. The groups at Visual Training for Tennis Clinics turned out to be half Pure Dextral (Serena, Andre) and half Cross Dextral (Roger) for instance in Phoenix we had 16 players tested, and it came out nicely 8 and 8, which helped with court assignments, in Atlanta 23 players came, and we had 13 pure dextral and 10 cross dextral. Now let's talk about how we test, and what the terms mean.

### Eye Dominance/Dextrality Test

The test:

1. With both eyes open and no squinting find an object in the distance or across the room.

2. Place your hands at full length away from you.

3. Make a small circle between your two hands and with both eyes still open find the object through the hole in your hands.

4. Close your left eye.

5. Do you still see the object? If yes, then you are right eye dominant.

6. Open your left eye, and close your right eye to confirm results. If you still see it with both eyes closed, then your circle is too big.

Some people are unable to close one eye for whatever reason, so you can use something to cover your eye as you do this. That's the first half of finding out whether you are pure or cross dextral. *Pure Dextral* people are right eye dominant and right handed, or left eye dominant and left handed, the purity comes from them being the same side. *Cross Dextral* players are left eye dominant and right handed, or right eye dominant and left handed. From my experiences with my players and out on the road meeting strangers, approximately 50% of the population are either one.

### Ben In Alabama - Video Analysis

In this video on my youtube channel, Ben whom I met in Alabama at a coaches workshop, volunteered and was the perfect test subject, because he did a great demonstration of trying to do like Federer. He had been trained to do it that way, because you know, Federer is the best at this right? No, he simply does what works for him, and Ben learned to do what works best for Pure Dextral players. Before the clip we tested him and found he was Pure Dextral. I did a few 'before' strokes, enough to see what his strokes really look like, not just one that looks bad. Then I explained to him that he can keep his eyes looking at a place halfway between the bounce of the ball and his contact point. You can clearly see that not only is he more relaxed, but he is also producing a more fluid swing, and I stopped briefly because his first shot doing the best strategy for him produced a very sweet contact with the ball.

### Pure Dextral Strategy

Pure Dextral Players will try out looking at a place between the bounce of the ball and their frame, and they can find their ideal place, then they will track the ball across their vision into the strings, maintaining a relatively still head during the process. I try not to say KEEP your head still, because it seems to produce tension that doesn't help the stroke. Instead I say ALLOW your head to remain relatively still.

### Cross Dextral Strategy

Cross Dextral Players can focus on the ball from the bounce into the strings and allow their head to be relatively still through the hitting phase of the shot, until they have to move to recover. Some people tend to start moving before they have finished their shot, so make sure you finish, then go.

### Benefits, Results, Outcomes

There are two main outcomes that you will gain from this, many Pure Dextral people tell me that it helps their depth perception. Both styles of players will hit many more balls in the sweet spot of the frame. You might also find yourself more relaxed and on balance for your shot. If you are Pure Dextral, you might also let go of the frustration of trying so hard to be like Federer, when their are other great champions that you can emulate for YOUR success. You can easily reduce the amount of errors in your game by a few shots per set! After many years of practicing as a Cross Dextral player, I now almost never mishit, it would have to be an extremely forcing shot for that to happen. Like Ben, you are more likely to play with less stress in your neck, and also make fewer errors, while also hitting more cleanly.

Nine

## How To Reduce Visual Distractions Without Yelling 'Focus'

*Keep your mind going in the right direction
and your life will catch up with it.
~ Joyce Meyer*

One of the most important ways to keep your mind on your match, is to keep your eyes inside the boundaries of the court. Once your eyes get interested in something else, other than your match, then you run the serious risk of losing concentration on your match. There could be some sort of disturbance or distraction happening on another court, someone fell, there is an argument or injury, or just some other interesting object in the environment. When you are on a main court and it feels like many spectators are watching your match, it's dangerous to get any sort of eye contact with any of those people.

The eyes are the window to the soul, if the eye is good, then the whole body is good, but if the eye is bad, then it all goes badly.

It's very easy to misinterpret a look from a stranger, so just don't look directly at anyone outside the court. My players are instructed to keep their eyes inside their court, and only on that which is important for them to see. Like the expression 'in one ear and out the other,' when you let someone's words simply pass right through you, you can also choose to let all non-essential visual experiences pass right through without thinking about them, but this is made more difficult when you get full eye contact, it's harder to 'Un-see'. Go into every match with only have a few things you are interested in seeing, the ball, the court, your racquet and your opponent.

### What Do You Play?

You don't play the opponent per se, you play the ball that they hit, and when any part of your minds CPU is being used up on other things not related to your match or the point, then you are distracted. The ball does not make anything personal, it's not emotionally charged, and it rarely takes a bad bounce, unless you are on a bad court. Clear those things out of your head, you can repeat 'only the ball,' 'only the ball' as a mantra, and also you can remind yourself to keep your eyes inside the court.

Of course, if you are playing in a beautiful location, on a changeover as a relaxation phase activity you can enjoy the beauty of your surroundings for a moment, but be careful to bring your eyes right back ready to play.

## Looking For Emotional Support

If you are a junior player, or any other player, please stop looking outside your match at the people watching you. A major mistake players make is looking outside for some kind of emotional support. You really are on your own out there, and you should know before the match whether you have the support of your team, or loved ones. Looking outside, looking to someone for something, that can distract away from your concentration for the next point. In fact, it can send you into a mental free fall, because the visual distraction you created, brought on thoughts that are not productive for winning a tennis match. On the other hand offering a quick smile to your team, and/or a glance that does not dwell can be a way to maintain connection with your people without committing your mind to the act.

It's common that when you gain eye contact with people, human nature dictates that we also often wonder what they are thinking, and judge that by the expression or even micro-expressions on their faces.

Vic Braden was part of a team that studied the effect of parent's micro expressions on the performances of junior players and found that when parents made bad faces, then players played more poorly. I'm going to assume that most parents don't think they are making bad faces, but often they are, because they have not learned how to manage their own nerves in their child's match.

## My Son's Experience

One thing I always did for my son was to stay very far away from the beginning of his match, during the warm up and the first game or two, then I would come a little closer, but try to find a place to watch from where I was not going to be in his direct line of sight.

## Team Matches

When I have played in team matches, I have sometimes asked my teammates not to stand in a place where they will be the last thing I see while I am serving or returning. In coaching high school tennis, I ask my team not to put their fingers through the cyclone fence and stand right up against it, because on the inside of the court, it can feel like that person is on your back.

We ask our off court teammates to stand a good 10 feet back from the fence, and not try to engage any lengthy eye contact with the player on court.

A few years back I had a player who was really having a tough time in her match, and she also had a certain personal issue that was plaguing her for a short time, but when her brother showed up to support her, standing directly behind the court, and trying to get full eye contact with her to show her he cared, she then went down the tubes. I started by explaining to him why that wasn't helpful and asked him to move to a corner of the court and stand in a shaded area, and also look in her general direction and only offer verbal support.

## Gamesmanship Ploys

Some opponents will use visual distractions to try to throw you off your game. They might hang their towel on the fence at eye level to change the uniform background view of the fence, or they might have some distracting behaviors that are intentional or unintentional, but still distracting like a weird toss behavior, ball bounces or a weird serve motion. They might also do some strange things when they return. You have to accept those things, but have a strategy to pick the ball out of those idiosyncratic motions. However, what you should NOT accept are when the opponent attempts to serve before you are ready, assuming you are playing to their normal pace. When a returner does something strange like shuffling their feet suddenly, when that is not a part of their normal return of serve preparation, that is outside of the rules. You can stop your match to let them know, and if they do it again, you can get an official.

On the other hand, anyone is allowed by rule to return from different positions on the court, and that is a good and smart way to create a difficult visual challenge to their opponent inside the rules, so again, you will have to accept it, read and react to it.

Many good players will come far forward to take the return, partly knowing that it can make the server feel pressure. Instead of looking at where you want to serve, you get distracted from that and start looking at them. It's vital that you look at the place you want to serve, rather than your opponent. I strongly recommend that you hit a very firm serve at the body on the backhand side to take time away from them when they do this, it can discourage them from this behavior, because the weakness in their ploy is that they make themselves vulnerable to the body serve.

## The 'Stink Eye'

Another issue that comes up is the bad attitudes of opponents, and how they use their eyes to scowl, intimidate, and try to make you feel bad. I recommend that you don't invite them into your mind, by bringing them into your mind, by giving them access to your eyes. If they are doing this a lot, give them just enough eye contact to be polite, but not enough that they can look right into your eyes to intimidate. As a good sport yourself, you wish for the other player to also be a good sport, and maybe you think you can melt them with your kindness, but they are not thinking that way, and they want to take advantage of any chink in your armor, so keep strong visual defenses up, while of course maintaining your classy great sportsmanship. My players have found this to be helpful. The player that uses this ugly behavior then will have no outlet for it. Sometimes that works against them. When you also always are cheerful and friendly to the player who is being mean and nasty, then you show them that they can't affect you. If you can't pull off cheerful and friendly, at least be civil in your behavior, don't allow them to drag you down, they will try to get in with your eyes. If you do all these things, you won't have to tell yourself to focus.

Ten

# Why I Don't Say "See The Ball, Through The Back Of The Strings"

*Don't believe everything you read on the internet.*
*~ Benjamin Franklin*

I occasionally receive emails or am asked questions on social media about articles or videos that players or coaches have seen on the web. One such article discussed whether Federer intends to see the ball through the back of his strings. I am using an article that was sent to me as an example and discussing some of the issues presented, but not giving attribution, because I wouldn't want that author to think that I am picking on them. Instead, this chapter will point to what seems like better teaching.

## Ideal Hitting Zone

There is an ideal hitting zone for your contact point between ball and racquet. Commonly, average players meet the ball too late, allowing the ball to cross their vision more than better players. Sometimes the ball even goes past their body completely for a shot that can be very tough on their elbow. Better players take the ball out front, where they can also deliver better leverage on the ball. Thank you to one of the major influences in this work, Jack Broudy, for showing that this is approximately 45 degrees away from you in front.

At one point, I obsessed with trying to make my contact point exactly 45 degrees away from me, but developed some tennis elbow, so then discovered that it's more approximate, and likely my ideal contact is slightly behind that angle.

With one handed backhands my experimentation has shown me that, the racquet arm at 45 degrees away from the front shoulder is nearly ideal, while in a two handed backhand, the triangle formed by both arms, as they contact the racquet at your hands, that triangle should point to approximately 45 degrees for maximum efficiency.

## Better Vision In Front

The most productive aspect of this contact point, is that you get better vision with less effort, and your leverage on the ball is better. So many aspects of your game will be positively affected by this concept. Also, it allows you to see the blur of the ball through the back of the strings, even though I don't believe that that one piece is crucial in visual skills.

Another benefit you will find is that it's easier for your head to be relatively still at contact, and your balance will not be under as much challenge. What you might find is that in order to achieve this, you will need to begin to see the ball sooner, as we have already discussed. There are other reasons why meeting the ball in front is better for your ability to focus, which you will also read about soon. It also, opens up an entry point to the zone which we will share from Scott Ford's work from Integral Consciousness in Sports.

## Benefits After The Shot

Another benefit of meeting the ball properly out front is that it reduces the angle, by which you will need to shift your gaze, to see the ball approach your opponent, AFTER you have finished your follow through. Biomechanically there is something great that happens out front and that's why pitchers and quarterbacks release there, batters hit there, hockey players and golfers also strike, and boxers punch at approximately 45 degrees.

## Why A Range Of Angles?

Another reason for saying that it's approximately 45 degrees in front is that different grips require different distances out in front to be successful. Western grips have the furthest forward contact, followed by semi-western. Eastern grips are better with contact maybe slightly behind 45 degrees, and continental grips will have an ideal contact that is slightly behind an Eastern grip, but ALL of them are ahead of the body for the most part. Strangely enough, when a ball gets behind you, it also works well to wait for it to be approximately 45 degrees behind you, and it's not had to flick it back using your iron chef backhand grip on a forehand shot pancake flipping skills.

## Moving Ahead With Your Eyes

After the hit, there is nothing wrong with allowing your eyes to jump forward to see your shot bounce, then track the rest of the way. What you don't want to do is compromise the hitting of your shot, the efficiency of it, by shifting eyes and head early. Finish your shot well, and maybe it doesn't come back, don't finish your shot well and maybe it goes into the net or becomes an easily attackable ball by your opponent. Doing the most with your shot, by allowing your eyes and head to be as still as possible increases the chances of that happening.

Eleven

# Why You Should Fine Tune Your Understanding Of Balance

*No one can see their reflection in running water.
It is only when it is still that we can see.
~ Zen Proverb*

There is a notion that for best vision of the ball players need to keep their eyes level and be perfectly balanced. However, when you look at top players at contact, you will often see that their head is often slightly tilted. Additionally, one of the very best tennis coaches I know, Doug King, teaches that players should be leaning ONTO the ball. In a vacuum of movement, without the requirement of hitting a tennis ball, your normal balance is predominantly upright.

**The impact of the ball and the racquet, through your arm and by extension your body weight, changes the mechanics of your balance.**

The force created requires a dynamic balance, or balance in motion. Ideally, you want to have a very slight lean toward the ideal balance point, where you can deliver the most efficient energy onto the ball. You lose some energy delivery when you balance yourself separately from the ball.

## Experimentation

A great way to experiment with this is to use a stationary ball, like Billie Jean King's Eye Coach, The Topspin Pro, or even a friend or coach holding a tennis ball out in their finger tips firmly (the best solution), until you find the ideal amount of lean. Doing this just enough allows for best leverage onto the ball, but going too far compromises your balance and vision while not gaining additional force.

## Court Position As A Factor

Another factor to consider when looking at the relative balance, level or tilted head and eyes is the court position of the player. When a player has been driven far back behind the baseline for a high deep shot, then it's only natural and probably ideal for their head to be tilted slightly back to see the ball. Conversely, a ball short and low in the court will require more lean forward, and a great slice shot on a low ball will mean that absolutely your head will come forward towards the ball. Incoming shots that are hit relatively comfortably, with plenty of time to get in position for ideal balance, posture and position, those are the shots that you need to find your optimum position for vision.

## Maximize Stillness, Maximize Focus

One thing that is required for focus, is that your body is relatively still, and when you look at the best players, they maximize what I call 'The Still Moment'. They are transition from the end of their footwork, into a momentary base, during which time, in ideal situations, their feet show almost no movement, except to rotate forward. In ideal ball striking positions, the player about to strike the ball has arrived just in time to have a still moment, marshal all resources and deliver and on balance blow to the ball.

**Having fully given an optimal amount of energy to the shot, in the next immediate moment, recovery, then preparation for the next shot begins.**

One of the very good old school instructions is to 'bisect the angle of your opponent's possible shots', I will add that as you begin to understand your opponent's tendencies, then you might also shade your positioning slightly in the direction of where they like to go with certain shots, or bait them into hitting something counter tendency. Where you move and the relative unpredictability of where you set up, changes the visual field for your opponent.

## Be Sure Not To Take It Too Far

It is however still true that you want to be relatively upright, balanced, and avoid excessive head tilt, and I do see players doing that from time to time. Recently passed legendary player and coach Dennis Ralston, did an amazing job with Chris Evert, getting her back to #1 in the world, and one thing he did was help her get back on balance. He did a simple exercise on her forehand where she would place her left hand on her forehead, while hitting the shot. Placing the hand there, immediately brings full attention to the relative position, balance and movement of the head. As you may have noticed, your eyes are connected to your head, and if you head is moving, then your eyes are moving also. Relative head stillness is critical to focused vision in the final stage of the ball's flight.

## Hand On Forehead

Try this the next time you go on court, hit a few forehands, then place your non-dominant hand on your forehead and notice how much tilt and movement there is with your head, while checking your relative balance. You can also place your hand on your opposite shoulder to check balance there as well. Your head, being about the weight of a bowling ball on top of your neck, can severely hurt the balance on your shot, and dramatically increase the stress in your body, as your neck, and the rest of your body struggle to keep it up. Probably, you will automatically make an adjustment to what you are doing after a few shots. The cumulative effect of being more on balance for more shots out of the hundreds you hit in a match will save you energy and errors.

### Next Steps For Mastery

After you feel like you have done that enough to get the experience in a few minutes, in between rallies, simply pat your forehead, to remember where it is, shifting your focus by being aware of your forehead, now you are also ready to do some backhands. It's even more awkward to try to hold your non-dominant hand on your forehead while hitting a backhand, so simply putting your hand on your forehead in between rallies restores the awareness if you lose it.

What are you noticing about your relative positioning to the ball? Are you closer or further from the ball? You may for the first time realized that you want to be much more precise in your final few steps to maximize the efficiency of each shot. The only thing to avoid is trying to be too rigid in your posture, or in trying to keep your head perfectly still or level.

Twelve

# How Your Legs Help Your Eyes

*Legs feed the wolf.*
*~ Herb Brooks*

An amazing thing happens when you ascend to higher levels of fitness in your lower body. As your leg strength, and your overall core and lower body strength come together, you can play at a lower altitude. When you play at a lower altitude, you can get your eyes down closer to your contact point on lower balls, which has a dramatic effect on your ability to see it more clearly, and to attack the ball. Conversely, when you play too tall, and the angle of incidence from the ground changes your ability to see it clearly as it comes up, and your head may tilt downward more than you need.

## Take The Challenge

Nick Bolletieri says that the 'athletic position' is one full head lower than standing straight. Try this, stand tall, and touch your neck, then get in a ready position where the top of your head is where your hand was when it touched your neck. How is that? You may have just discovered that you need more fitness in your game to get your eyes lower with the ball.

## Upward Explosion

Nowadays more players are launching themselves way up to hit high balls, and this must be very well timed to allow for the eyes to have an adequate amount of stillness to still focus well on the ball. It is ill advised for intermediate players to attempt these jumping shots, and there may be some dubious returns from those who can execute it well. A great question to ask is, does a player gain an advantage by hitting from a place with no ground reaction force by hitting further forward in the court? Another great question is whether they mitigate taking a defensive posture that they would have taken by moving further back to take the ball while their feet could still contact the ground? Finally, would the player be better able to recover for the next shot, if they did not have to land, and then move? Studying this might be difficult, but it's worth considering as a player whether leaving the ground a few feet on purpose is worthwhile. Of course, there are many times that players lift off of the ground do to the sheer combined force of the ground reaction, and their racquet head speed. Jumping and lift off are on the same.

Thirteen

## Why 'Hungry Eyes' Are Not The Solution And What To Do Instead

*If trying hard isn't working, try softer.*
*~ Lily Tomlin*

I'm here to make vision of the ball easier, playing tennis easier, advancing through levels just a matter of time and talent. If you, however, are addicted to trying harder, because you think it's difficult and are unwilling to change, then this book is not for you. I have worked with many Type A personalities, and some Type A1s.

When I and my students have gone about the work, or learning to take it a bit easier, we have also often branched out into taking their drive down a notch in life, allowing things to flow better for them.

It was important for me to learn this for myself, in order to be able to show the way to others. I still have moments of Type A behavior, although not A1 very often. Type A, is a psychological term for how driven a person is, and Type A1 is the most driven. I'm writing for those with a growth mentality, who will take this knowledge, explore what resonates with them, realizing that due to the wide range of visual differences that exist between people, that some concepts will fit perfectly with you, and not compute at all with someone else. So, if a particular chapter does not compute, please read it, but then move on to one where you find more value. Type B personalities might not even know what I am talking about here for them.

### Trying TOO Hard

Nearly 100% of the tennis players, when they come for a first lesson are using their eyes poorly, or at least not close to full efficiency. The most common behavior I see, comes from an attitude about life and how to succeed. For most people who come to tennis, there is a sense I get from them, that if they try hard enough, they will learn how to play. In reality they are trying way too hard.

**This over the top effort creates stress, and the anxiety that comes with it actually clouds their minds from seeing what will help them play better.**

Their eyes and mind are full of effort. The problem there, is that there is an amazing amount of work that your visual ability and your brain do PASSIVELY, unthinking, without you having to try at all. Recent studies have shown that when you gamify your learning to make it fun, then you can learn complex tasks up to 80% faster, according to Greg Patton (no relation), USTA National Coach. Of course, you need some physical effort, in fact you will need effort that will take you pretty close to your maximum heart rate, but visually and mentally, you can do much better by NOT trying so hard to see the ball.

## The Symptoms Of Over Trying

There is a thing I call 'hungry eyes'. Players come out on court and they are half squinting, they have tension around their eye sockets because they are forcing themselves to focus. Their internal dialogue says, 'focus, focus, focus'. Or they are operating out of some internal deficit believe that they lack something, and have to try hard to overcome. I say, 'play tennis', but they seem to try to analyze every move, because they have to remember, and tell themselves how to do it later. Instead, the most common thing that happens at the end of my first lesson with a student, when I ask them, 'What was the most important thing you learned in this first lesson?', they say, 'to relax'.

**When you look at the top players in the world, the higher you go, the more relaxed they become.**

Many aspiring champions, trying to break onto the tour, and become a regular in the top 100 have failed to do so, because of a lack of relaxation, because their inner drive creates tension in their body and in their eyes. The worry about outcomes of matches, finances, and what comes next gets in the way. They carry an anxiety that clouds their judgement, restricts their movement, and does not allow them full clarity of the play situation. Serena Williams when at the height of her game had this ability to become one hundred percent immersed in the situation, she had an ability to flip an internal switch to come from behind in matches on the toughest stages. Between Djokovic, Nadal and Federer, their switches are mostly on at all times, but if their internal switch of calm awareness where to be switched off against one of the other two, you can be sure they are not winning. Every top champion admits to feeling nervous at times, and we have discussed why that is a good thing.

## Practical Steps To Seeing Better In Your Lesson and Play

What is the practical thing to do here? Come to the court in a relaxed state, let go of tension in your body, let your eyes go soft. Have soft focus. Get warmed up, and increase your physical tension to an optimal point, where you have the ability to move explosively, while still free of excessive tension, allowing your eyes to be soft. Imagine receiving a gift. The ball is the gift, put your hand out to receive it. When someone hands you a gift, do you grab it from their hand, or do you stay where you, in quiet expectancy to hold it? It's in the grabbing, and frantic moving to the ball where errors are made, so this concept is more about the attitude of receiving and reception skills are probably not taught by tennis coaches nearly enough.

Our minds are so interested in the sending skills, the strokes, the hitting, the footwork, the effort, things we can see. Most people can't see how a player sees, but with training, you can. When we dismiss most of the issues that create tension and over trying, opening our eyes to welcome the ball, our mind, our brain rather passively puts us in position to receive it well. Of course, it takes some time and experience for you to learn this well, but if you get out of your brain's way and allow the most powerful computer on the planet to do what it does naturally, it finds the ball. Your eyes and mind get you where you want to be for the best possible shot.

## Play, Not Work

Another common thought that I dispel in lesson one, is that we can let go of the idea of working on our game. It's an oxymoronic statement, 'working' on our 'game'. We 'play' games. So play around with your game, this refers back to the research shared by Greg Patton. Have a playful attitude, and you will find that you learn things more quickly, by playing around with the concept. Experiment, have fun, discover how to do it. You will also see more clearly what is happening. You don't play with hungry eyes. Playing comes with soft eyes.

Instead of making tennis another outlet for work in your life, learn to play better. This forms the baseline for toying around with the concepts in every chapter after this one. Have fun with it, and you will find that it's easy, and you may also discover more joy in your play, because then you will find recreation, and a release from the tension of daily life. Enjoy a different attitude about the game you love. So take a scan of your body, and sense where you hold tension, prepare for play by getting more relaxed, rather than more hyped up. Let the ball come to you and allow yourself to move smoothly too it. Simply receive the gift of the ball with enjoyment.

Fourteen

## How To Move Beyond Past Experiences By Developing Visual Skills For The Present And Future

*We are the sum total of our experiences. Those experiences — be they positive or negative — make us the person we are, at any given point in our lives. And, like a flowing river, those same experiences, and those yet to come, continue to influence and reshape the person we are, and the person we become. None of us are the same as we were yesterday, nor will be tomorrow.*
~ BJ Neblett

Everyone owns their own visual experiences, but many were handed some through poor teaching. Your best thinking brought you here, and now you might have to leave behind conventional wisdom of seeing the ball. Visual training is the new frontier in every ball sport.

One piece from the BBC Brain Special that seems to indicate the need for many years of visual experience, was the case of a man who had lost his sight at age 3, then 40 years later received stem cell treatment on the damaged part of his eyes, thus regaining his sight. According to doctors, the process was a complete success, and his eyes regained full anatomical function. The man who regained his sight, let's call him Dan, when he was being driven home from the hospital, was terrified of the road signs overhead on the freeway. Each one it seemed to him, that they were going to collide with the roof of the car. Everything that moved seemed to be some type of threat for Dan.

He could not recognize his children by sight even after a few years had gone by, but he could recognize them through touch. Ten years later, he was still confused by dark shapes in his peripheral vision. He still can't easily differentiate between a person, a tree, or a shadow along the ground. Dan never fully regained his facial recognition ability, and still uses a guide dog to keep him safe. The conclusion was that Dan can see, but his brain had become very busy wiring his other senses more completely using a larger part of his brain's overall function, that his visual processing was compromised in the long term.

## How Does This Apply To A Tennis Player?

It takes a bit of time to develop enough experiences with the ball, that it won't seem like an emergency when it comes. It takes still more time, to continually rally the ball back and forth, maintaining eye discipline to continue, for many shots in a row. Quite a few year more are needed, to be able to read and react quickly, to any particular shot from your opponent. And still more to develop a set of contingencies in regard to what shot you will hit next.

It would seem that this experience and the discovery about how the brain works to develop meaningful perceptions and especially moving objects would have a bearing on how we experience one of the most challenging moving objects in sports, the tennis ball.

One of the most difficult visual tasks, if not the most difficult, in all of sports is hitting a baseball thrown by a Major League Baseball pitcher. A tennis ball coming at faster speeds can be just about the same level of challenge mitigated only by the greater distance, the fuzz on the ball, and how it slows down additionally after the bounce. Even so, returning serves over 125 M.P.H., or more, that are expertly placed is nearly impossible. The much wider variety of behaviors of a tennis ball interacting with polyester strings and tennis courts creates a much tougher challenge to be able to read and react.

## Ball Recognition

One of my most common coaching phrases is 'on a ball like that, do this...,' as no two shots come the same way, but certain types of shots require a completely different skill. A different approach needs to be taken for a short slice shot compared to a deep topspin drive, or a huge looping heavy topspin ball. Ball recognition is something to begin with early, and that supports the idea that players will do better with early exposure to tennis. This is not meant to encourage early specialization in any way, in fact the exact opposite. A wider variety of sports experiences enriches the visual lexicon of experience.

Tom Stow, one of the greatest teachers of tennis, in the history of the game, was expert at drawing out other athletic and artistic experiences of his athletes, to create analogies that created a deeper understanding of how to play tennis.

Sherylle Calder, Ph.D a preeminent visual training consultant in the professional sports world, and has tested 100,000 athletes finding that no two have the same strengths and weaknesses says, 'people need to climb trees and fences, walk narrow ledges to challenge balance and have a wide variety of visual experiences to be well rounded visually.' So you can also stand on one leg, play with catch and throw different kinds of balls, play video games and challenge your vision with reaction time and reflex drill equipment like BlazePods, and watch yourself play on SwingVision. These are best practices in learning any ball sport, and it mainly applies to the visual experience paired with kinesthetic and the kinematics of the other player.

## Discover Perceptual Issues with Video

What if we could slow the ball down so that players can actually see what is happening. We can! Everyone who has a smartphone has access to slow motion video which allows a coach to show a player exactly what is happening. What you can look for is how are players responding to the ball. Can you track the moment they made a maladaptive move based on delay, anxiety, or not being fully present?

There is very little to argue, when using slow motion video, from the perspective of the player, when they can see plain as day, exactly where they made contact with the ball, then you can back track to root causes.

In that setting, using technology, a collaboration between player and coach occurs, to understand what triggered or delayed the move. Solving the perceptual problems in large part, starts right there, with the outcome of the interplay, between the ball and strings. This builds the pairing of the kinesthetic with the visual. I have just purchased 10 used Flip Cameras, that are very inexpensive and have a USB attached so that I can plug them right into my computer. I film every lesson now, and upload onto my YouTube channel, so that students can look back at what they learned in a lesson.

## Start At The Origin

It's been said start where you are, use what you have, do what you can. Start with your contact point, discover what was the largest or most easily solved problem you had, in getting to an ideal contact point. Stay with that issue, until you reach a certain level of mastery.

Visual awareness of ideal contact points is one the most critical fundamentals to master. It takes many years of experience to develop a complete catalog of visual experiences and learn the myriad of moves to become complete at dealing with any kind of ball. Djokovic is now the supreme example of this, while Federer formerly held that mantle.

## Conclusion

There are no absolutes when it comes to learning or teaching visual skills and understandings, because each person has a unique way of seeing. Understanding that you are unique is important. Consider that when you are a new player every ball can seem like an emergency, even so bring your awareness to your contact point and you will be surprised and how much faster you can learn than others. As you begin to rally, see the ball coming out of the opponent's frame. Then be patient as you take the highest priority training items from this book and slowly work them into your game. It's going to take some time.

Fifteen

## How To Effectively Model Strokes, Learn Without Hitting A Ball

*By three methods we may learn wisdom:
First, by reflection, which is noblest;
Second, by imitation, which is easiest;
and third by experience, which is the bitterest.
~ Confucius*

People largely learn tennis through imitation. The mind's ability to clearly and accurately see what is really happening, both in the modeled behavior, and in their comparison of their own behavior is essential. Knowing really what is happening with the ideal technique, and the performance by the student, removes a considerable amount of interference in learning. In communication theory, there is the message from one person, the channel, and what is received on the other side. Clarity is key.

**If the message is not clear, or the channel muddled, then it's even more difficult for the hearer to correctly interpret the information, and the same analogy holds true with the eyes.**

During the Cybervision era, video tapes were made of Stan Smith and Chris Evert, who were known as the paragons of perfect technique at that time. There was great data that people who watched those videos would go out and play better tennis the next time out, without additional instruction.

### Imitation: The Sincerest Form Of Flattery

It's been proven that one of the most effective ways to learn a new movement is simply to have it modeled for you. When someone successfully and somewhat repetitively demonstrates a movement, your brain picks up on the cue. Choose wisely whom to mimic. If you do not have very large biceps, I don't recommend watching Nadal. If you are 6'5, I wouldn't recommend watching Diego Schwartzman. Generally it's true that you would want to find someone with a similar physique, but also a mentality of play that you are capable of playing. Pair that with rehearsal and the kinesthetic feeling of going through that motion, and you can begin to learn it for yourself.

## The Importance Of 3D

Watch great players, but be careful. Watching players in real time in 2 dimensions does not allow you to see every movement in the plane in which it's occurring.  Watching in person is better, while viewing from different angles. Watching in super slow motion helps your mind to truly identify what is really happening, as opposed to remnants or archaeological term.  Example, people feel like they see Rafa rolling over the ball, but when he really hits it well he is hitting completely through and his follow through goes amazingly forward before his forearm turns over.

**A minor mishit in the lower third of the frame can make the frame and forearm of the player distort, and it then appears as though there was an intent behind that, then you get comments like 'that's a windshield wiper forehand'.**

The same is true with a well struck slice ball.  The frame takes a dip at contact, forced slightly downward by the impact of ball and strings, the observer then thinks they see a chopping of the ball, when in fact the intent of the player was to knife straight through the shot. So, in visualizing, you want to be as accurate as you can and not pay attention to residual images.

Seek out the very best images, watching in slow motion and from many angles for a better understanding of what you want to do. Then film yourself doing it, looking for the ONE big variance, and start with that ONE thing to work on, before moving on, or work on the first part of the breakdown of the shot, to see if that also solves other issues on the timeline of your stroke.

Sixteen

# Why You Can Ignore Early Specialization Gurus

A new meta-analysis, however, indicates that the 10,000 hour rule simply does not exist. As Brain's Idea reports, authors of the new study undertook the largest literature Survey on this subject to date, compiling the results of 88 scientific articles representing data from some 11,000 research participants. Practice, they found, on average explains just 12 percent of skill mastery and subsequent success. "In other words the 10,000-Hour rule is nonsense," Brain's Idea writes. "Stop believing in it. Sure, practice is important. But other factors (age? intelligence? talent?) appear to play a bigger role."
~ Rachel Nuwer

The reality of what is best for your longer term development, health and maintenance of your visual acuity for sports and life is having a wide variety of visual experiences. Contrary to the 10,000 hour rule of 'time on task,' which would seem to indicate or at least be interpreted as doing the same thing over and over again. That would be practicing tennis. It turns out in peer reviewed studies, that 12% of your competency, comes from practice. The other 88% comes from your age, intelligence and physical talent level. It's only common sense that a person with a severe developmental issue will not likely ascend to the top of world class tennis even with 10,000 hours.

**Coaches in every sport acknowledge a player in the game who lacking size, strength, speed or some other factor, have '[name of sport] Intelligence'.**

Yes, putting in the time is important, and for some who are less talented, they might need to put in more time, but not in the way you might think. To maximize your tennis intelligence, you will want to look at it in different ways, using overtraining of your visual system to enhance abilities that can make up for any relative lack of pure talent. I have seen plenty of good tennis players who happen to be overweight, and it's their superior ability to read and react to the first ball which allows them to compete with players more fit to play the game.

**If you have all the talents, and still want to go higher, you also need this wide variety of visual abilities and challenges.**

Dr. Sherylle Calder is one of the world's leading experts on visual skills as they apply to sport, her story is amazing, and her research sheds like on the best practices for maximizing visual ability. Sherylle's story is amazing because she practiced in nearly complete isolation from players of her same ability, because she grew up in South Africa during Apartheid, and the South African sports community was isolated from international competition. She was a talented field hockey player, who practiced by herself, without teammates or competition to push her to new heights.

**She tried every different way to play with the ball, using walls, uneven surfaces, and every other different way to see how the ball behaves.**

When she finally left South Africa to pursue world class play, she amazed her peers, and would often be asked: 'How do you do that?' or 'How did you know that was going to happen and where to be?' Sure, she simply could be talented visually, but it seems to indicate that she became more intelligent about the ball. She became a force in the sport and after her time on the field, she then devoted herself to the study of visual skill development. Now having tested 100,000 athletes, and seen that no two athletes have the same capabilities, she asserts that everyone should do their best to have the widest variety of visual training experiences to build up these capacities.

Seventeen

## How To Facilitate A Wide Variety Of Visual Experiences On A Tennis Court

**Rolling, Multi Bounce, Any Way You Can Hit** - If you are a tennis person who dogmatically states that every child needs to play with an adult regulation yellow tennis ball and take every ball on one bounce, then you are missing out on opportunities to give younger and younger players an opportunity to develop their tennis vision and intelligence. With players six and younger, allowing for a brief time of rolling a red ball, then making it bounce, followed by allowing only one bounce, and then transitioning all the way through to yellow balls, is a great way to develop an achievement mindset.

**Balance Exercises** - Balance and Vision are linked, and having different types of ways to challenge balance are good. Walk on a ledge, stand on a dome cone, balance and hop on one foot then the other, etc. Unstable surface training, might not be a great thing for players who want to be fast. Even though they challenge balance, they also reduce mobility in the lower body. A narrow, stable surface is preferable.

**Off Balance Drills** - I have a drill called Plyo Groundies - where a player hops over two cones and then as soon as their foot hits the ground a feed is made to the opposite corner of the court. This sends players off balance, running fast, and they will need to recover their balance to some degree to make the shot.

**Reaction Time Training** - There are many ways to train reaction time without any technology, and it's easy to eye ball some improvements, but the next two tools are pretty amazing, because you can add different elements to the training.

**Blaze Pods** - Are an amazing device of which I am an ambassador. I use these every week, and sometimes many times in a week. My players have made dramatic shifts in their reaction times to the incoming ball, but practicing not only visual decision making, but also reaction and movement drills. Use this link for 15% off. They are rechargeable electronic light stations that respond to touch, and can be programmed in multiple ways for many kinds of uses.

**Q-Balls** - These irregularly shaped balls are great, because I find that some reaction balls are simply too aggressive and can lead to injury as players make sudden movements that can lead to injury. These balls also have numbers on them, which allows you to create games. I recommend using two of them, one for each hand.

**Juggling** - keeping multiple objects in the air at the same time is a great way to develop your peripheral vision, and thus your tracking ability.

**Hanging Upside Down** - There is a phenomenon called 'Fighter Pilot Brain,' which means that those who have this ability or have developed it on their own have the ability to know where they are spatially in reference to the ground. Most commonly elite gymnasts have this and are amazing at knowing where the apparatus is in their mind without having to see it directly. It's a great idea to spend a little bit of time hanging upside down on a bar, or some apparatus to develop this capacity. This will help you on those balls where you are way off balance to hit, like retrieving and extreme wide ball or great drop shot.

**SwingVision** - this is a relatively new AI driven app funded by Andy Roddick and James Blake that does real time data in your match. Simply filming yourself to watch later is a huge piece in the visual training system, because you can reflect back on certain points, putting together how you look from the outside, together with how it felt to hit the shot, and how it looked from inside you. Adding real time data, like where the shot actually hit compared to where you thought you hit it, and the relative speed of the ball informs better decision making and awareness.

**Gamesense** - this is an app that is in late stage development. I have had the chance to experiment with it, and I am on the development team. The app uses occlusion in a novel way, in that the clip of a server hitting the ball suddenly ends, and at that point you are asked to predict the location of the serve. This is an amazing technology, because the better you can learn predictive cues from the subtle differences in how your opponent sets up and swings through to their shot, the better you will be at everything that comes after that. This should become available in 2021.

**Video Taping** - as stated earlier, the simple act of video taping and then watching it back will help you quite a bit, but there are a few factors to consider. The best view to watch is immediately behind you at eye level, because then you will see more similarly to what is realistic. SwingVision, however operates best at the top of the fence, so for playback and visualization it's very good, but not completely ideal. In training, its a great idea to film from the side and also at a 45 degree angle ahead of you, because different aspects of technique will begin to show up in different planes.

**Drone View** - looking at the match purely from above should not only be fun, but also educate you better on the true depth of your shots in a chalk talk format, you will see the court from a clipboard view, and that's always interesting.

**Chalk Talk** - I don't often get out my clipboard with a tennis court drawn on it, but when I do, there is bound to be a player who sees for the first time with a forest view, instead of staring at the trees. When you can look at the court globally on a small format, the geometry seems easier for some people to process visually. Sometimes the magic is in the pairing of the images on the board and the reality on the court.

**On Court Walk Through** - This is another way to bring spatial awareness, but in a full body experience. When I teach System 5 to my players, we take a tour of the zones around the court, and I also pair the relative backswing lengths, then we practice each size backswing as we go back through the zones. This allows players to identify which zone of the court they are in, and make the appropriate backswing decision, and then we also teach some of the mitigating factors that will create exceptions to the general rule, like when the incoming shot is very fast, makes you run a long distance, or is very high or very low to the net and how that affects your backswing.

**Blow the Whistle and Freeze** - if you are coaching, having players stop right where they are on the court in the middle of a point, simply asking them 'what do you see?', can be extremely illuminating. When done a few times in a set, players can begin to see their relative position, and doubles teams can see openings given or to use to win or lose points. When they stop, they can actually see better what has happened.

What do you see? In general, this is one of the best questions to ask yourself and others. What do you see in your opponent to exploit? What do you see in your game that you can improve right now? What do you see in the patterns of your opponent's play? Keep in mind, as Craig O'Shannessy of Brain Game Tennis says, "You are the second most important player on the court. What your opponent is doing is #1". Take mental visual notes about what is happening on the court, so you can answer the question, 'What is going on here in this match?'

**Where, Where, Where** - Where is the ball? Where do I want to make contact? Where do I want to hit it? These are my new questions in 2021. This has been a bit of a breakthrough, since 'where' runs through the faster pathways of your visual system, and defeats overthinking.

Eighteen

# Why Is Eye Dominance Fundamental Knowledge? Using The Eye That Does Your Most Seeing

> In general, eye dominance goes along with handedness. In other words, lefties' left eyes are more likely to be dominant while righties' right eyes are likely to be dominant. But there are many exceptions to this rule. For example, according to one study, about 35% of right-handers and 57% of left-handers are left eye dominant.
> ~ Troy Bedinghouse, OD

Things get even more complicated if you're ambidextrous (a switch hitter), or use different hands for writing and throwing. According to one review, 28.8% of left-handers and 1.6% of right-handers by writing were inconsistent for throwing. For this group, it's almost impossible to correlate handedness and eye dominance.

## Dominant Eye Does Most of the Seeing

Your dominant eye gathers the bulk of the information about the ball. Everyone has a dominant eye that processes information to the brain a just a few milliseconds faster than their non-dominant eye. "The dominant or sighting eye also guides the movement and fixations of the other eye." (Kluka, 1991). The combination of eye and hand dominance has been a topic of a recent study of golf putting (Steinberg, Frehlich, & Tennant, 1995). It was found that those who are pure dextral (same eye dominance has their hand dominance right eye/right hand, left eye/left hand), are best advised to focus on the space between the ball and the striking implement. This would seem to empower the use of peripheral vision. Cross dextral (right/left, left/right) people perform equally well attempting to focus directly on the ball, or at a place between ball and striking implement.

**In plain English, if your dominant eye is on the opposite side from your dominant arm, then you will be more successful focusing directly on the ball.**

If your dominant eye is on the same side as your dominant arm, then you may be best advised to focus at a place between the final bounce, and the contact with the ball to allow for greater use of peripheral vision.

Thus, 'keep your eye on the ball,' might not be the best advice for everyone.

## Discover Your Eye Dominance

To discover which is your dominant eye, locate a small object at least 20 feet away. Using a lone tennis ball on the other side of the net is a good way to do this. Stretching out your arms to full length, make a tiny opening between your hands, just larger than the ball. When you can see the ball in the small space with both eyes open, then close your left eye. Do you still see the ball? You are right eye dominant. With right eye closed, if you are seeing the ball with your left, then conversely you are left eye dominant. It's important to form the hole in your hands and center the ball with both eyes open, so that you will naturally select your dominant eye, do not attempt to sight the ball with one eye closed prior to centering the ball inside the small space.

## Your Nose is in The Way

Once you identify and intentionally are using your dominant eye to 'see' the ball, while allowing the non-dominant eye to help provide the depth perception, and three dimensional cues, your ability to read and react to the ball may increase. Be mindful that if the bridge of your nose is between your dominant eye and the ball, you can turn your head to aim your eye more in that direction. It can be helpful for you to turn your head so that both eyes can see the action. An example would be a left eye dominant player hitting a backhand volley.

**If their head is turned too much to the side, then the non-dominant eye will be forced to be responsible for tracking (sighting).**

Using the non-dominant eye for tracking may lead to more errors, and fewer well centered balls on the frame, regardless of how much time you have to see the ball. This may explain why people make errors on slow moving balls and get frustrated at missing an easy ball, simply because they were looking with the wrong eye.

Now that I have taken this material on the road as a guest clinician, I have received plenty of great feedback from clinic participants, some of whom found it to be a revelation. It seems that the population is approximately 50% each Pure and Cross Dextral. The pure dextral players seem to be the best helped by a novel approach to seeing the ball, which causes me to think that they have been underserved. So if you are a coach reading this, you might find some wow factor for your students.

## Training Eye Pairing, Dominant and Non-Dominant

One way to improve your overall vision is to exercise each eye separately. Get a comfortable patch to place over one eye at a time. Be sure to practice at a very low challenge level for only a few minutes at a time. Start with 5 minutes of covering (occluding) your non-dominant eye, then do 5 minutes of covering your dominant eye, looking only through your non-dominant eye. Then finish with 5 more minutes of hitting with both eyes open. This is a great thing to do for the final fifteen minutes of practice, because your eyes may be too tired to continue. Of course, you can try simply closing one eye, but it's extremely challenging to keep one eye closed for a full five minutes.

Nineteen

## What Are The Visual Considerations For Each Shot?

## The Serve

*The Serve Will Always Be The Most
Important Shot In Tennis.
~ Tennis Maxim*

The visual skills of the serve are fairly simple compared to all other strokes, but there are some intuitively wrong actions people take with their eyes. Ultimately, the most important thing you can do, is allow your eyes to see the contact point, for as long as is naturally possible. The serve is also the most important shot for you to be able to hit your targets with precision. A serve that was supposed to go to the body, but instead is a ball to your antagonist's forehand 'wheelhouse', might find you in instant trouble from a strong or winning return. The varied deliveries that you give, mixing up speed, spin and location gives you a visual advantage, because the opponent may begin to read your average serve.

**Over the years of playing many tournaments and coaching, I have been surprised at how predictable people can be with their serve.**

Even the 100+ MPH first serve that does really well in the first few games, becomes less daunting to the opponent, if that's all you hit, and even less so, if you seem to hit it to one place quite often. The three serves you must own are, a slice serve wide in the deuce court, a flat serve into the body on both sides, and a topspin or kick serve to the backhand on both sides. Building in more serves will make you more effective. If you are able to make the ball go wide to the forehand, and high to the backhand, then you have a very nice unpredictable range.

### The Toss

Many new players, and some seasoned ones, intuitively believe that some advantage is gained by watching their toss from their starting position, all the way up, as they lift it up following it with their head, neck and eyes all the way to the top. All of that head motion, causes the eyes to also move, it also changes your balance, because your shifting head is actually pretty heavy.

**Instead, simply look up to the place you will be tossing.**

With your eyes lifted to the contact area, scanning that small field up at contact, there will be great benefits: 1. You will be better aware of the location of your ideal toss. 2. You are likely to have a better awareness of your balance. 3. Your eyes will be more still. The act of serving can seem a lot less chaotic. 4. The accuracy of your toss can improve, as your vision of the field you are tossing into, becomes more easily seen.

## Lifting Your Head

It's a best practice to lean ever so slightly back with your chest, to get your head tilted slightly back, directing your eyes at the ball. Standing straight up, tilting your head back only at your neck, is not desirable, because it will affect your balance, and it makes your neck vulnerable to injury.

## Checking Targets

It's always a good time for a reminder, that your best training will establish your targets, in your imagination. If you must take a peek at where you want to serve, make sure that on subsequent serves, you also look in other places in the service box. Also, you can use your scanning vision, to locate your target without looking directly at the place you want to serve.

**When your eyes are up at the toss location at the moment of contact, the target will either be out of your vision, or in your extreme periphery.**

Your peripheral vision will not give you great eyesight on the bullseye. Some level of trust will need to exist for you, in your ability to see the target in your mind, to hit your targets, and that will come from regular serve practice. As you improve, your ability to notice the subtle changes in your hand and wrist position at contact create different serve locations, speeds and spins, You might not need to look over at targets in the service box again, because they are all stored in your mind. Watch a professional tennis player, and try to guess where they are serving based on their body language, especially their head and eyes. Good luck with that.

## Be Predictably Good

It's important NOT to obsess on being unpredictable, even though some unpredictably will give you an advantage. One great example is that when you are playing someone and you have a great advantage in speed, so you want to serve most of your serves to the outside corner, and wide on a shorter angle, so that you can get your opponent off the court and moving.

**You will give up a bit of mystery, because you probably want 80% of your serves out wide.**

You will hit just a few deliveries into the body, or into the T to mix things up a bit, keeping the other player honest. The same applies for a situation where the other player is the faster player, wanting to make you move all over the court. You will be best advised to serve to the T, or the body on the inside part of the court, so that you can keep them in the middle for the return. Again, the element of surprise is not on your side as a visual tactic, but the geometrical advantage gained is worth it. Also, some matches come down to the fact that only one or two of your serves are effective on the day, so it doesn't make sense to mix things up too much, if you are missing serves, or they lack the necessary sting you want to make them work. So don't worry about being predictable, if the situation shows you that it's not on the menu today, to balance that out, you do want to through in just enough of the other serves to keep the opponent from completely grooving their returns.

Twenty

# The Return Of Serve

*The Return of Serve is the second
most important shot in tennis.
~ Tennis Maxim*

The return of serve is not a groundstroke. The origin point of the shot, makes it unique in many ways, as it comes from relatively the same place in singles, but in doubles there can be enough variance to change the rhythm of the shot. The very best returners of all time, successfully return approximately 80% of all serves into the court, so that means 1 in 5 are not returned. The visual challenges behind returning serve are the most difficult in the game, for a shot you will see at least 4 times every other game. In an average match you might see 80 to 100 serves, so that gives you some time to start to read your opponent. You are facing someone who gets to put the ball right where they want it, and hit it as hard as they can.

**In most matches, the first serve is the fastest shot on the court.**

To compound this, serves also have the greatest variances in spin, because not only is it hard to match a topspin serve where the server can launch all of their athleticism upward to the ball and create approximately 5,000 RPMs or more, jumping above shoulder height, and sometimes above the level of your head. Slice serves that curve significantly away from you, or into your body are also a challenge, and no other shot behaves the same way. It's imperative that you learn to read and react.

**Best Reactions, Time Savings Are Essential**

You must read the ball at the earliest possible time, taking in the wholeness of the way your opponent attacks the ball, and begin to look for tendencies. Occasionally, you meet a player that reveals their intention for where they plan to serve. They might stand a certain way, take a practice stroke, look at their target, have a little twitch, or some other 'tell'. The story goes that Andre Agassi has never told Boris Becker, that there was a little thing that he did right before serving, that showed Andre what Boris intended to hit. Agassi beat Becker 10 out of the last 11 times they played including matches at the US Open, Indian Wells and Wimbledon! Return of serve was the key to those wins.

## Returning First Serve - Defense First

- See the ball out of strings
- Immediate Shoulder Turn With Eyes Still Forward
- Track ball to the bounce, paying full attention
- Very Short Back Swings
- Meeting the ball squarely for the flattest possible shot.
-  is the best option for the fewest errors.
- Slicing or chipping the return is the next best option,
- because you can also take some pace from the ball
- Hitting Excessive topspin is a bad idea and will lead
- to more errors than are necessary
- 

## Returning Second Serve - Think Attack

- Shift Mentally Into Attack Mode
- Move Slightly Forward to Return
- Go at the Server With the Return
- Create a Severe Angle
- Approach the Net
- Drop Shot

**Here are a couple things to look for your opponent to do that can give away their shot:**

1. Looking at their target
2. Making a grip adjustment
3. Adjusting their feet a certain way
4. Taking a practice swing
5. An involuntary movement in their body
6. A pattern one type followed by another
7. A certain serve in a certain situation
   - A. First point of a game
   - B. 30-all
   - C. Break Point
   - D. Game Point

In the cutting edge of visual performance training, all the top trainers are referencing Kinematics, or reading the physical performance tendencies of players. There are many new technologies that allow you to start to have better reaction time decision making in regard to the placement of the shot. We have already mentioned Blazepods, SwingVision, and GameSense, and future editions will strive to keep an updated list of the newest technologies, although it can't be stressed enough that low technology solutions can take you quite far. The strategies in this book being among them.

## Study Your Opponent, and All Opponent's Carefully

If you want to be the smarter visual player, then you have to take notes mentally on the different things you see. Look for things that are different, because it's very easy to see the different things, when most of the other behaviors are the same. This partly explains why Pete Fischer taught Pete Sampras to wait until the very last moment to hit the kind of serve he wanted, thus making Pete's serve one of the best disguised in the history of tennis.

## Build In Unpredictable Tics, Think Poker and Bluffing

You can also use this in the converse to fool your opponent, as there are things you can do, to throw your opponent off, making it more difficult for them, to able to read your serve. Whatever you do, don't overthink it. For instance, I like to look at my target, then serve to it a few times, then I will look at a place that is NOT my target, to see if my opponent is looking at where I am looking. Try not to make it too obvious. I then will save that for a time when I really need it, like down 15-30, break point against, or with my first game point in a serve game I desperately need to hold.

You have to practice your serve a lot, if you are going to make serves to your target without looking directly at it. One way to begin using this strategy is either to first look at your target, then look at another place where you are not hitting, or vice versa. This way the other player will have to decide which one you are hitting, and that can take their mind to the slower thinking mode, which we will discuss more in future chapters. The more you can get them to think about which serve you are about to use, the less likely they are to simply read and react.

Twenty-One

# The '+1 Shots'

*It's OK To Win In The First Two Shots,
But It's Not OK To Lose In The First Two Shots.
~ Craig O'Shannessey*

It's true that most of the content of this book applies to what happens after serves and returns are hit. However, now that we have taken a closer look at the first two most important shots in tennis, lets turn our attention to the +1 shots. Yes, a sudden shift in attention is very important, because of the relatively quick changes that occur in the complexion of the point from serving or returning to the next ball that comes.

The most important aspects of making the next shots are being decisive and having maximum reactivity. The situations can be fluid, and visually you will learn to shift quickly from reacting to defense to being decisive about offense. The default position if to react to defense, since you don't want to make errors on balls that are not attackable.

**One of the very fine dividing factors between good, great and elite level play is how effectively a player takes advantage of balls to attack without chipping in forced errors.**

The key stat that is enhanced when you begin to put more pressure on opponents with more balls is that you will force them into more errors. You may also marginally improve the amount of winners that you get, but we will call those happy accidents. Errors, forced and unforced still account for two-thirds of all point outcomes.

### Serve +1

Serving then going into the next shot means that you start with the most serene and controllable moment, into the most chaotic. The shot that most often is hard to predict is the return of serve. It can be so often mishit, mistimed, over or under reacted to, often the returner doesn't even know where it is going. What you need are very well trained contingencies. Perhaps a particular serve will get you a nice forehand 70% of the time, a sharply angled one 10%, a high deep one 10% and a ball to your backhand 10% of the time. I have simply made up some numbers here for comparison, your actual breakdown will vary. So if this is true, then most of your training will be for the 70%, but you will also need to spend a little time preparing for the other three likely scenarios.

**As you can see, it's paramount that immediately after completing your serve, your full attention goes to the returner to read what is coming out of their frame.**

You must first prepared to play defense, but ready to shift into offensive mode as soon as you see that the ball is where it needs to be for your attack. When it is not in that zone, then you will shift to your other mode of playing the ball in a particular zone. You need quite a few If This, Then That's in your game. You also have to be ready for that ball that is barely returned and drops barely over the net for a drop shot. What is your play?

## Return +1

The return, appropriately so, is the most defensive regular shot you will hit on first serves, and can be one of the most offensive shots on second serves, depending on the server. Your top priority is to see that ball into your strings, making a good enough shot to stop the chaos. On most balls, when you can get the ball deep at the server, or deep cross court, you buy your eyes more time to see the ball. But when you drop it short, the opponent can take precious reaction time away from you. When you think of returning as something that takes pressure away from your visual system, then you start to approach it in a different light. When the opportunity presents itself against a weaker server to attack serves, thus putting your opponent's reactivity or decision making under pressure, then you can gain a foothold in the point or force an error right away.

Immediately after making your return, and simultaneously with recovering, you have more time to follow your shot, and break down into a great stance at the bounce of your ball, ready to read and react to the Serve +1. Keep in mind, the most common rally length is 1, followed by 2, followed by 3. So if you make your return and the next ball you have a huge advantage over those who lazily miss returns or second shots. Your top priority is to play defense first, but also be ready in some instances to take advantage of opportunities to attack. Leaving shots that can be turned into offense on the table, can prolong a point needlessly. It's ok to win the point in the first two shots, but it's not ok to lose it.

Twenty-Two

## **The Groundstrokes**

*80% of people who play tennis simply want to rally.*
*~ OnCourt OffCourt*

Visual issues of groundstrokes seem subtle to most people, but fundamental to the Visual Training Player. It's pretty common that players will be much better on one side than the other. Many people can relate to having a good forehand, but not such a great backhand. Surprisingly and somewhat painfully, players with good backhands often have relatively weaker, less predictable, or more error prone forehands. To the player with poor backhand, that seems like a shame. The most important core explanation for this revolves around eye dominance, but there are other factors of stroke making, not covered in this work, that can play into the differences between one side or the other.

By now you have taken the dominant eye test, and possibly now you will have an a-ha moment. I'm left eye dominant, and my forehand was not as good as my backhand, until I learned how my dominant eye affected the shot. There are two ways to go wrong with using your dominant eye. First, you might not use it, instead relying on your non-dominant eye.

**Interestingly enough, first I had to improve my backhand, in order to understand how that affected my forehand.**

My backhand improved, when I learned to turn my head forward enough to sight the incoming ball with my left eye. For years I struggled to see the ball well enough, because the dominant eye can't see past the bridge of the nose. Second, you might use your dominant eye too much and turn it toward your other side. My forehand was very unpredictable, because I would turn my head so much to 'keep my eye on the ball'. It wasn't until my thirties that my forehand became a weapon, when I learned to keep my dominant eye forward, and use the tracking skills of a cross dextral player. I focus on the ball from the bounce into the strings, but not with the same amount of head movement in the last phase. Now in my late fifties I rarely mishit or put any balls in the net due to so many years of working on my visual skills.

The bottom line is this. Once you know your dominant eye, make sure you intentionally use it to pick up the ball, it does most of your seeing. As the ball approaches, know your style, pure or cross dextral strategies. Execute your visual strategy, with minimal head motion and you will hit much cleaner on your weaker side, and perhaps improve on both sides as I did.

Twenty-Three

# The Volleys

*Those seen dancing were thought mad, by those who could not hear the music.*
~ Nietzsche

The most important issue to resolve for people that affects their vision of the ball at the net is anxiety. Even for players who are seemingly proficient in their volley mechanics, the reduced amount of time to see and make contact with the ball can be a source of overreactions.

**Players generally play an anxious game of tennis from the baseline, and when they get to the net, subconsciously they calculate that they now have even less time to see the ball at net.**

In order to cope with what seems like not enough time to see the ball, they do everything they can to speed up their reactions, and that is the source of many missed volleys, and a lot of cumulative nervousness. The solution is to start with how much time there really is, making the most of it.

### There Is So Much Time

When I first start teaching the volley with a student, we begin with the time/space continuum. I help them to understand exactly how much time there is to see the ball, and it's actually more than enough. We discuss briefly how people start to freak out at net and that time seems to speed up.

**So, we say There Is So Much Time. Then we say it again very slowly one word ever second, There... Is... So... Much... Time...**

We then will do a little volley rally and each time we make contact with the ball we will say one of the words. What that helps players to realize is that there was plenty of time to say each word, and there was quite a bit of time between each contact of the ball. That creates some mental calmness and space to get the other objectives done, and they get progressively more difficult. So, I stick with the volley rally until we get into a very calm, easy rally. Then we start to get a bit more technical in our approach.

## The Ball Out Of The Strings

Seeing the ball out of the other player's strings is even more important at the net, but there is a subtle difference in the performance for volleys. At the net, I don't discuss pure and cross dextral, as there is not really time to focus on the ball, instead almost all the attention goes to the frame on the other side of the net. After contact, simply tracking the ball into the frame leads to some amazing improvements in getting the ball centered in the strings, which is half the battle to hitting great volleys, because then you don't have to try as hard to finish. Another common issue then arises, the fact that a player will repeatedly miss the center of the strings, hitting the same place on our near the frame. This stems from a perceptual issue, in that they think the ball is higher, lower, closer or further than it really is. This can take a few moments to resolve as the player has to take stock of where they are missing on the frame, realizing that they have to do the opposite of what feels natural. In a few moments of overcorrecting, they can find their new contact point.

## The Next Step In Challenging Players

Make sure you go from hitting only forehands, or only backhands to hitting forehands then backhands back and forth while remaining calm, picking up the ball out of the strings each time. Strangely enough, it's more important to look at their strings than it is your own, and your peripheral vision is actually quite amazing for centering the ball.

## Close In Volleys

Starting at the T, or on the service line, volley forehand to forehand, and keep coming one step forward after each shot. The shots should be fairly soft, but firmly struck and with the best possible accuracy to go right to the other person's forehand. As you get closer and closer, the reflexes of the drill are increased, just because being closer takes away time.

**There will come a moment when you get a certain distance from the net and your anxiety will ramp up, and you will find it difficult to get all the way to the net.**

You will recoil and want to move backwards. Instead, calm down, slow down and stay where you are a moment, then proceed forward again. I do this drill with all my players 3.0 and above. We also then make some attempts to trap the ball between our two racquets, and while it doesn't happen in the first attempt, or even the first few days of trying, eventually it does happen. Once you can stand about two feet from the net with your partner the same distance away, having a volley rally, then you are ready. The amount of time that it takes for the ball to go back and forth from that distance is the same as if someone hit a screaming forehand passing shot from the baseline. The drill will make it much more likely for you to realize you have plenty of time to make that volley.

### Alternating Volleys

The same drill above has a next logical progression for more difficulty and real life application. One player should hit forehand volleys, but they should alternately make the opponent hit forehand, backhand, forehand, backhand while also moving forward. Still accuracy of shot to keep the volley rally going is essential. If you can hit it into your opponent's racquet, then you can also hit it precisely in between two players on the other side!

**The secret sauce here is that many people practice forehand and/or backhand volleys in isolation, but they don't often practice going from one to the other repeatedly, with the same target for both shots.**

Sometimes, you play a doubles team, and one of the players has a weak volley, this trains you to pick on that from either side. Other times, you play a team and they have four solid volleys as a team, but one or both players miss when they go from forehand to backhand or vice versa. You are now trained to pick on that. As you will see, moving from side to side creates a new visual challenge, and heightened anxiety level is possible. Continue to see the ball come out of the opponent's racquet, before you take this to the final stage.

### Butterfly Volleys

In the final iteration of this series of visual challenges, one player will hit straight ahead and the other player will hit across, and if you diagram it, it looks like a sharp butterfly. One player hits their forehand to the other player's forehand, and their backhand to the other player's backhand. The other player continues the rally by hitting their forehand to the backhand, and their backhand to the forehand.

**Stick with this arrangement and gain some mastery before changing to go the other direction.**

It's smart to allow the better volleyer to do the cross court shots first, as it's slightly more difficult to hit. Continue to move in. Now, doing this you make yourself better trained so that a player can't use the same tactic against you, and you can keep them challenged while they are challenging you and may the better trained player win. I'm pretty sure it will be you, and people will say, 'how do you do that?'. If you like them, tell them.

### High Low Volleys

One of the ultimate confidence builders for reading and reacting to volleys is the high low volley drill. It's likely you will need an experienced coach, or expensive ball machine to do this drill, someone who can feed balls accurately is very important and it's not an easy feed. Start by having the feeder give you pretty easy low forehand volleys, followed by high backhand volleys, then increase the tempo until it's pretty challenging. Then go back to a slower tempo, but make the feeds where you will take a crossover step and recover to ready position, before taking a crossover to the other side. Move to low backhand volleys followed by high forehand volleys.

**I like to do this in either the deuce or ad court box, if you have a certain side you play, practice in that side.**

The targets are the center line or the singles sideline, because you can get the ball past another net player easily if you hit those, at the very least you create an opening in the court. Once you are 75-90% accurate at hitting near those lines, then have your feeder stretch you out to the maximum you can move and reach for these shots, but not further. What you will find is that your dynamic range of movement for volleys will increase dramatically and your ability to read and react. Finally, for the super advanced players, one ball directly at the volleyer, or a low lob for a soft overhead, can be a surprise that is a great way to protect against those things as well. I recommend that for strong 4.5 players and above.

## The Romanian Volley Drill

With a partner start on the service line at the side T standing cross court from each other. Volley one, two and on the third shot start moving to the middle of the court, both of you should arrive at the center T at the same time, then continue to the other side T. The addition of lateral movement with ball placement to a moving target will help you to be able to hit spots on the court even as opponents move. Your lateral movement will also add a new visual element to the challenge.

Twenty-Four

## **Lobs And Overheads**

Lobs and overheads are under practiced, so before we get into the visual issues, it's important that you add regular practice each week, even if for just a few minutes. There are not a lot of mysteries when it comes to the overhead visually, but a few general concepts can make things a lot easier.

1. The default position is that you should want to **take the ball out of the air**. The advantage gained by doing this takes away time and space from your opponent. So if you lazily take overheads off the bounce because it seems easier, then you are giving up an advantage.

2. You must **decide quickly** if you are going to let the ball bounce either because the lob is too high, too low, or behind you. It's almost impossible to change your decision from allowing the ball to bounce, to taking it out of the air as the visual system will become confused, and this is when you see some of the most embarrassing overhead errors.

3. **Choose your target before you swing**, and commit to it, no matter what opponent's do. One of the best things you can do as a lobber is to move toward the opening, and try to make the overhead hitting change their shot. You can reduce how effective they are, or even cause an error. So, as the overhead hitter stay committed to your target and hit it well, because you will still be on offense, even if they have a chance to return it.

4. The best targets are to the **opposite side of the court singles sideline in doubles**, or down the middle. For singles going to the deep corner opposite where your opponent is can be a staple. Avoid the feeling like you have to be tricky.

5. **It's not a serve** and there are good and bad things about that. Your opponent is trying to give you the world's worst toss. But, you don't have to hit it into the service box, and you don't have to hit it from the baseline. If you conservatively aim for a firm shot to the open court, then you will win 80% of those points easily. If you pitch in too many errors, then you wont be that successful. Keep in mind sometimes people do make perfect lobs, and they also can suddenly hit an amazing shot now and then off of an overhead, so you will never win 100% of those points.

Twenty-Five

## How Does The Time/Space Continuum Play Into Vision? How Being Fully Present Improves Perception

*Since time is a continuum, the moment is always different,
so the music is always different.*
~ Herbie Hancock

The time/space continuum plays at once a complex and a very simple role in our ability to experience our vision in the present. In Scott Ford's book, *Integral Consciousness in Sports*, he outlines some very important concepts that play heavily into how we perceive time and space with our eyes and mind. Scott created a timeline of perception, and presence. First, he defines being fully present, as a time when the absolute present meets the flowing present in our minds. Being fully present is a key indicator of 'The Zone,' its one of the most commonly reported characteristics of the Ideal Performance State. There are two elements of the present, the flowing and the absolute present, and when the flowing and the absolute two converge, then there is opportunity to enter the zone easily.

**The absolute present, is your seemingly permanent self, who you are, which changes so slowly as to seem permanent.**

Think of a massive tree, when you look at it each day, it seems to be the same, but everyday something about it is changing, leaves or needles fall, and it's growing, but it seems to be unchanging, that is analogous to the absolute present. The collection of experiences that make up who we are, one after the other, moment to moment, that is our flowing present. Gradually dead leaves and needles fall, and are replaced by new. The flowing present can be expressed through reading these words: now, now, now, now.  Each time you read the word now, it was NOW, but the first occurrence came before the other three. While reading those words, your absolute and your flowing present are connected, but if you get distracted by another thought of something in another place or time, then that presence is interrupted. So, just like when you read, your zone time is limited by your ability to pay attention. Attention, presence these are things that can be developed and practiced. Now let's put it all together.

## The Process of Presence

The first phase of the process of presence is understanding that everything you SEE is in the PAST. By the time your eyes pick up the sensory input, allowing the information to pass through either your dorsal or ventral pathway, the event has already happened. There is an inviolable .04 seconds of reaction time, and maybe longer depending on your capacity to react. No amount of training will shorten this finite amount of reaction time. During that .04 your brain has you fooled into thinking that it's the present. In the next phase, everything you are DOING is in the PRESENT. When you are running to the ball, then that's what you are doing, this is what you know very well, it's the first and the last phase that people are not as much aware of and how it affects their presence.

## An EVENT You Are Moving To IS In The FUTURE

In Tennis that event is mainly the contact point. The key is to be fully present, having your flowing present and your absolute present together, in your experience of each phase. Our brains fool us into thinking that was has just happened is in the present. It's painfully simple to understand, but it takes time and practice to apply. While we can sharpen ourselves to become much more engaged with the present moment. We can be more fully present in our actions and with our interactions with people, there will be times that we slip into the past, or have an urge to wish for the future to arrive early, or to be in another place entirely, sometimes it's any other place.

## Fully Present With The Past

The moment you see the ball coming out of your opponent's racquet, it has already occurred, and there is a delay in the time, between the actual event, and the time you process it, seeing it in your mind. What is most important is to be fully present with our experience of what we are seeing?

## Present With The Present, Not Getting Ahead, Or Stuck

When we make our first move to the ball that does happen in the present moment and our kinesthetic experience does not take much process time in our brains. Even so, many players habitually carry with them a shot from the past that invades this moment, or they are anxious for the future moment. Being fully present with the present experience is vital to the outcome of the shot.

Finally, we are moving to a place, in the future where we will meet the ball, staying in time with that moment, is the final piece of the timeline for that shot.

Rather than rushing, getting ahead of ourselves helps us to execute the shot we want. It's not a paradox to run very fast, while being very patient, waiting for the moment to strike, and that is part of becoming an advanced to elite player.

## Compartmentalizing the Process

After each shot, making a clean break from that particular shot, puts it in the past. We don't want to drag that past with us into the present, or moving to the future. No matter how good or how bad our last shot might have been we want to be fully engaged in preparation for making the most of the next shot. Then we can stay fully engaged in the match moment by moment.

## Two Main Sources Of Physical Errors

Since learning this time/space continuum issue, I have come to realize that there are two main root causes mentally and emotionally that lead to physical errors. Immediately upon teaching the concept of being fully present with the ball, I have seen with new eyes the errors my students make. Surprisingly enough, many of the visual errors made come from the associated anxiety, confusion, distraction, self-criticism, lack of confidence of not being fully present, having their minds busy on something else. Many people are working so hard to be ahead of things, or to make up for something in the past, that they can't wait for the ball to arrive, so they flinch. Some of my determined, conscientious students like to keep their minds busy, beating themselves up for their poor performance.

**It's as if people think that, 'If only I criticize myself enough, I will perform better'.**

Still others approach the hitting of a tennis ball like a checklist of items, that are performed in sequence in their mind. Still others use a medical model to diagnose what went wrong. Perhaps the worst question a player can ask is 'How do You do it?', the studying of the process of hitting a stroke mentally with traditional thought leads to 'paralysis by analysis'. Their minds are so busy with these activities, that their eyes can't see clearly what is happening. While their brains are so busy, the ball is still moving and they are stuck in their head, living in the past with instructions given previously, so they can't really see the ball very well in the present.

## Focus on Place, Experience Time

The exercise that Ford, a founding member of the Evolutionary Sports Collective, espouses is to bring your visual attention to one place and learn to wait. Imagine an ideal contact point by putting your hands in front of you like a mime making an imaginary wall. Now, place your racquet against that wall for forehands and backhands, high, medium and low. You might discover that the range of motion creates bit of a convex in front of you. Now, when the ball approaches, track it from the opponent's frame, but focus on your barrier.

**Pay attention to whether you allowed the ball past your barrier or not.**

Taking the ball a bit early is fine, but late can be a problem. Say, 'yes' when you meet the ball at the barrier or in front, and 'no' if it gets past it. This can bring you into an amazing awareness of waiting for the ball to arrive, and while focusing on that, some other things happen in your mind and movement of which you can take note. Recently, I have started to say 'now' every time I hit the ball, this seems to me to be a personalization of Scott's discovery. So, my mind is not even on the barrier any more, but on the simple awareness of the contact point.

Ultimately, visual skills are about finding your best methods for tuning into what is real about the balls flight. Taking ownership of learning how to get yourself in ideal position, at the ideal time, to create the most efficient force, direction, and spin on the ball for the shot you want. It's an endless pursuit. Now onto the next one!

Twenty-Six

## Why Is Ball Recognition An Evolving Problem? Train And Care For Your Eyes

*Time is an equal opportunity employer. Each human being has exactly the same number of hours and minutes every day. Rich people can't buy more hours. Scientists can't invent new minutes. And you can't save time to spend it on another day. Even so, time is amazingly fair and forgiving. No matter how much time you've wasted in the past, you still have an entire tomorrow.*
*~ Denis Waitley*

The problem of ball recognition is reaching greater and greater levels of complexity since the introduction of polyester strings, and the influx of players 6 foot 5 inches tall and above who can hit very high bouncing topspin serves.

I noticed something recently while at the Indian Wells Professional event featuring WTA and ATP players. Players outside of the top 20, and increasingly so as their rankings are lower, seem to not be quite as highly skilled at early tracking of the ball. One the particularly difficult conditions in dry climates is the more unpredictable flights of the ball with less moisture to slow the ball. This leads to more off-balance and inefficient shots. Roger Federer is perhaps the greatest model of this type of ideal performance of arriving at the ball in ideal position and balance, while players like Nadal and Murray have had many struggles at Indian Wells.

### Time Savings with Timely Reaction

Players who are inside the top 100 in the world may take a closer look, no pun intended, at how they are training their eyes, reactions and movement for better performance on court. My feeling from experience is that one of the major barriers to overcome to play 4.5 and above is tracking heavily spun balls.

Most of the positive results that I have seen or heard, in learning about athletic visual skills, seem largely to be anecdotal, so I am relying on your faith and a little collaboration with trial and error thrown in for good measure.

In my research, there was not one conclusive study to support an enormous gain in performance from vision training, but as Albert Einstein famously said, 'Not everything that counts can be counted, and not everything that can be counted counts.' Very few iron-clad conclusions can be reached in this field, and that's why after a brief foray into the research, I will be discussing more tricks of the trade from experienced coaches.

## Healthy Eyes are Essential

I have almost always been blessed with having great vision. There was a time however, when my health had taken a turn for the worse, and with it my ability to see with great clarity. In spite of the natural talent of great vision, I have had to go to great lengths and it took years to use my eyes close to the top of my ability.

Early on in my research, Duey Evans from Texas shared a video with me from an eye doctor, who stated that the first step in developing any kind of program is to check on the health of your eyes.

If the eyes are not healthy then some type of intervention needs to take place before moving onto challenging training. When my eyes were not healthy, I had lost some of my visual abilities. When I regained full health, then my eyes returned to their former ability. In this book, I will share many of the visual exercises and theories which I learned in my pursuit of training myself and my tennis players.

Almost every sport has visual cues that must be attended to so that the athlete can respond according to training. It must be noted that sometimes the visual stimuli that come in through the eyes to the ocular nerves, then can be transmitted straight to muscle nerve tissue, creating an immediate response, according to the level of training the athlete has assimilated.

Twenty-Seven

# Which Physical Exercises Strengthen My Eyes? Do The Eye Muscle Workout

There are some very specific skills related to the muscles that control your eye position and focus. In practicing, challenging, and performing the below exercises, if you find that you don't feel well while doing them, stop immediately, and schedule an appointment with the appropriate physician.

## Convergence

The ability to turn both eyes inward is important. The better you can do it and shift your focus will help you do a better job with focusing on the ball in the final stage of flight, after the bounce.

*The Exercise:*

Take a pencil or similar object with small ending in hand and extend it a full arms length away. Slowly, and I do mean very slowly, bring the tip of the object toward the bridge of your nose, allowing your eyes to turn inward, while maintaining focus. If you begin to see double vision of the end of the pencil, slow down and correct until you see it as one object again. I found that this was extremely difficult without my glasses, but once I put them on, it was still challenging, but I could do it. With the pencil against your nose, it wont be easy to truly focus, but at that stage keep single vision will be difficult enough.

## Sideways Tracking

The ability to see objects moving vertically across your vision, or even while your head is moving slightly.

*The Exercise:*

Find an object with the smallest character you can read. Place it at arms length, turn your head from side to side, but don't allow your head to go so far that you can't see the object with both eyes. Keep the character in focus, if you find that it gets significantly blurry, or you feel dizzy, nauseous or any other symptom, stop immediately. If all is well you will be able to keep reasonable focus on the small character or font.

## Vertical Tracking

Tracking objects up and down can be more difficult that side to side, and can lead to errors on high or low balls.

*The Exercise:*

Repeat the same exercise as Sideways Tracking, up and down.

## Peripheral Vision Test

Although targets in your peripheral might be best managed by relying on your imagination, adding more periphery to your vision, can make that more effective.

*The Exercise:*

Look straight ahead. Put your arms out and your side, wiggling your hands, can you see them at 180 degrees away from each other, or 90 degrees from straight ahead with no peeking? Now move your hands backward, the further back you can do still seeing the movement of your hands, the better. If less that 180 degrees, it may also be a good time to see a doctor.

Twenty-Eight

# What Do Visual Researchers Say Are Hidden Capacities Of Vision? Reconciliation And Imagination

*Our uniqueness makes us special, makes perception valuable — but it can also make us lonely. This loneliness is different from being 'alone': You can be lonely even surrounded by people. The feeling I'm talking about stems from the sense that we can never fully share the truth of who we are. I experienced this acutely at an early age.*
*~ Amy Tan*

Research clearly indicates that there are nearly zero cookie cutter answers for visual training from one athlete to another.

According to Kukla and Knudson, 1997, **'Vision may be the most variable and selective of all the senses. Attempting to observe fast movements that occur in sport places great demands on human vision.'** Our eyes work with our brains, and also circumvent parts of our brain in some instances. When working with the brain, our eyes send information, which then creates a three dimensional representation in the mind.

**Both eyes working together, create fusion of an image, sequence, and/or flow of events.**

Athletes must make an effort to attend to their performance, or the eyes will naturally move throughout the field. Thus the importance of ideal teaching cues, directing where and when to look, how to see are important to helping players discover subtle performance enhancing skills. When athletes give full attention, or allow an object to gain their attention, this is a conduit to fixation on the object. Learning to be fully present with the visual experience is the universal outcome that can lead to better performance.

## Our Brains Reconcile 'The Blur'

Fixation is necessary for best possible focus, especially of a moving object, as our focusing ability is limited to 3 degrees in front of us (Kukla, 1991). The same is true when reading well, your eyes will keep the letters within that narrow focal point. Three degrees is approximately the wide of your thumb at the end of your outstretched hand. On a tennis court, this is extremely demanding to maintain the ball within that 3 degree band, instead, there is a better way. In reality, when you read a word or a small phrase, all the other words appear slightly out of focus in your peripheral vision.

**The problem is that fixation is extremely tiring, and we often fixate at the wrong times and for too long.**

Underrated is our the ability of our eyes and mind to reconcile vision of the blurred fast moving object. If you don't learn anything else from this book, this idea of the mighty power of the eyes, brain/mind to process the trajectory of a streaking ball is way better than we give credit.

Part of the reason tennis players are the best readers in school, when compared to players of many other sports, is the relatively small size of the object they are tracking from 70 to 100 feet away from them. If compared to a font size it would be very small around a 6 font or smaller when on the opponent's side of the court.

### The Use of Imagination

Because the area of focus in the visual field is so small, the ability for an athlete to use their peripheral vision is essential. The advantage of peripheral vision is that the processing speed of tracking a moving object is very fast compared to any other type of seeing. Using peripheral vision in tracking the ball, also allows a player track their relative position in the play. They may also have enough brain power 'CPU' to visualize a target to hit to, prior to execution of their shot. As Styrling Strother asserts in 7 On Court Strategies, 'the target is in your imagination,' because your eyes are with the ball.

**The research proves this out that only a small percentage of your visual experience actually comes through your eyes at this moment, most of it is already stored in your brain.**

Of course, the ability to perform at the highest level of execution requires many hours practicing the imagery, knowing the environment, the geometry of the court. Some of the highest forms of praise given to athletes are: 'always knows where they are on the field, aware of where they need to be,' 'seems to know where the ball is going before everyone else on the field,' 'doesn't chase the game, lets it come to them'. In many other sports, becoming fixated on the ball or target can lead to a loss of attention to the peripheral vision necessary to execute a play. Inability to use the full field of vision can make a football player vulnerable to blocks, and other interference from the opposition. A tennis player might not notice that their opponent has snuck into the net, or moved a few feet inside the baseline altering their position on court to change the rhythm on the next exchange of shots.

Tennis players are best advised to fixate or focus on the ball from the bounce of the incoming ball into their frame, since at that time their body most often will have come to a relatively still position, and the peripheral vision tasks are complete. Once the ball is struck, peripheral vision tasks resume, tracking the outgoing ball.

Twenty-Nine

## When Do You Have A Lot Of Time To See The Ball? How The Ball Slows Down For You, Or Not.

*The thing about being a lifelong gamer is that my eye-to-hand reaction time is faster than average. I actually went on a website that tests your reaction time and verified this to my satisfaction.*
*~ Arthur Chu*

### Ball Interaction with the Air and Ground

Another very important shift in vision may take place upon the ball bouncing on the ground. I say 'may,' because when a player is on the run, they might not be able to focus at all, since the body's parasympathetic nervous system will not allow the eyes to focus. More than one-third of the time you have to see the ball occurs after the bounce. John Yandell's Advanced Tennis Research Project reported years ago that the ball slows down considerably from the opponent's hit, until it bounces on your side, mainly due to air resistance. Gravity also plays a role in slowing the ball down.

**Once the ball has hit the ground, the most dramatic slowing of the ball occurs, and it loses approximately and additional 25% of its speed.**

Because of the friction of the court surface, depending on what kind of spin is on the ball, it will slow down less or even more. Finally the ball continues to slow as gravity and air pressure continue to work to slowing the ball. In this final phase of its approach, after the bounce, we have enough time to truly focus on the ball. As the ball nearly reaches our strings it will slow to its lowest speed just prior to impact.

### Eyes Fully Informed Early

Some of our problems in seeing the ball may be explained by our use of the eyes in less than an ideal way. Most commonly on court, I see players who have not scanned for the ball out of the opponents frame, and are surprised by its arrival, they report that they try to pick up the ball somewhere along its flight.

**Others try too hard to focus on the ball the entire flight, and thus 'blank out' at the wrong time, and become extremely frustrated that they missed a ball that they tried so hard to keep in their pinpoint vision.**

This may explain why some people hate slow or high balls, because by the time the ball arrives, they are at the end of their ability to focus and may lose vision in a variety of ways at a crucial time to see the ball. I have found it easier to make better contact on higher slower balls when only focusing from the bounce of the ball on my side, then into my racquet. Focusing from the bounce also requires seeing the bounce of the ball, which is the second most important moment in tennis after the contact point itself, the finalizing of the prediction of contact point comes largely from seeing the bounce of the ball. When we use this skill it will be even more helpful when playing on an uneven surface. So use out this variety of visual skills, and try not to overthink it, the transitions come very easily if you don't try too hard.

Thirty

# Why Are Sleep And Recovery A Fundamental? How To Perform Closer To 100% More Often.

*Sleep is the single most effective thing we can do to reset our brain and body health each day -- Mother Nature's best effort yet at contra-death.*
*~ Matthew Walker*

## Effects Of Sleep On Visual Performance

There are many peer reviewed studies that show a wide variety of negative effects on visual attentional performance from losing only one good night's sleep.

## Tunnel Vision

Poor sleep within an 18 hour window can lead to Tunnel Vision, where more of your vision is directed to the very center, reduced awareness to all surrounding awareness. This might be interpreted as a good thing, but it means that you will have less awareness of where you are on the court, and where you need to hit.

## Interference With Flow

Performance deficits on visual tasks during sleep deprivation are due to higher cognitive processes rather than early visual processing. Simply put, your brain has to work harder to process when you lack sleep. Sleep deprivation may differentially impair processing of more-detailed visual information, which means that you will experience uneven ability to concentrate, finding it harder to enter a flow state. 15%-20% of car crashes are caused by sleep deprivation.

## Loss Of Attentional Control

A Study of 18 year old college athletes showed no significant difference in the ability to play powerfully, but did show a decline in attentional ability, especially reaction time. This could be tricky, because physically the player can feel normal, and not account for the fact that they have a lapse in concentration brought about by lack of sleep. This only after only missing one good night's sleep affecting performance.

## Socio-Emotional Issues

Athletes might be lesson expressive and impaired in their ability to recognize emotion in coaches and teammates. This might be cause for concern with teams that have team chemistry issues. A lack of sleep can make players less responsive to detecting visual cues in micro-expressions, body language and other non-verbal communications.

Athletes may also over react to perceived visual threats because the amygdala is negatively effected.

These ideas are not yet proven, but this new field of study has some early indications that there is some validity to these notions. My opinion is that many times these things can be true, but also you will find athletes who have an amazing capacity to perform well, even when fairly sleep deprived. As a general rule, everyone is going to get along better when they are getting enough sleep, also able to read the cues of their doubles partners, and other teammates.

## Caffeine

Caffeine works to block the receptors that would send signals to you that you are tired. It does not do anything to solve the problem of fatigue, it simply fools you into thinking you can continue and thus push past warning signs. In recent years caffeine use has increased, especially among young people, due to the wide diffusion of caffeinated beverages advertised as energy drinks. Caffeine does however aid in attentional ability in a serving of 75 mg, but higher levels do not significantly increase performance. The problem becomes over arousal after consuming more than 75 mg, so that any additional attentional control is mitigated by the jittery reactions that it creates. Studies do indicate that habitual coffee drinkers can tolerate up to 400 mg without a major decline in performance, and no habitual drinkers up to 200 mg.

## Caffeine and Reaction Time

The positive of caffeine is that the mental part of reaction can be enhanced, but the actual physical reactions don't show any significant difference. However, when people are under the weather, having a case of the 'two o'clocks' or working at night, caffeine can be a great intervention.

One strong cup of coffee is about equivalent to a 30 minute nap to reduce driving impairment, but taking the nap will actually provide the needed rest.

## Caffeine and Sleep

There is an effect on sleep by daily caffeine intake, so while caffeine seems like it could be the solution to some short term effects of a lack of sleep, taken regularly it seems to affect sleep negatively, so it's far preferable for the athlete to consume the minimum amount for their enjoyment. Not only does caffeine intake affect sleep quality, but also creates more daytime sleepiness, which can make it very tough to play a 2pm match in the heat.

The most-documented effects of caffeine on sleep consist principally of prolonged sleep latency, shorter total sleep time, worsening of perceived sleep quality, increases in light sleep and shortening of deep sleep time, as well as more frequent awakenings. Rapid Eye Movement (REM) sleep is less. REM sleep is a stage in the normal sleep cycle during which dreams occur and the body undergoes marked changes, including rapid eye movement, loss of reflexes, and increased pulse rate and brain activity.

Human sensitivity to the effects of caffeine on sleep is variable and its exact basis is still debated. A 2016 systematic review of research on coffee, caffeine and sleep concluded that individuals will respond differently to caffeine based on a variety of factors, including age, sensitivity levels, regular coffee and caffeine intake, time of consumption and genetic variability.

Thirty-One

# The Effects Of Environment and Recovery On Visual Acuity

*Practice does not make perfect. It is practice, followed by a night of sleep, that leads to perfection.*
*~ Matthew Walker*

The poor physical state of your body, can have a direct and negative effect on your vision and your reaction times. When you are playing in abnormally low temperatures, have not had enough sleep, are not fully recovered from a hard workout, or even worse are suffering from the effects of overtraining, then you are at risk for not being fully sharp. Your ability to see and respond with the precision you want can be diminished.

## Low Temperatures

The famous science TV show, Myth-busters, which was filmed 15 minutes from my house, wanted to prove whether it was true that you can be 'slapped to your senses'. The interesting application for us is that since they couldn't legally get someone drunk for the experiment or have them using illicit drugs, they did something else. They exposed the test subject to temperatures in the 30 degree range for a period of time, did some before and after mental and reaction time tasks, and found that performance was diminished dramatically in colder temperatures. The cool part was they found that being slapped in your face, creates an autonomic responses that sharpens the senses. So, if you are feeling drowsy and not alert, trip a little slap on the face.

## Sleep Interventions

In the last chapter, we dug a little deep in the research without really giving solutions, except that excessive caffeine intact seems NOT to be the answer. Recently, I have started to pay much closer attention to how long, and with what quality I sleep. Part of this has been aided by wearable tech that measures these things for me. So whether you get a Whoop, an Apple Watch, a FitBit or a Garmin or some other brand, shop wisely. There is a trade off in how much you invest, for how good the quality of the data you get. I have found that with even a slightly dubious measurement, over time I can start to see patterns of having slept better one night because of the way I prepared for bed. We have already covered many reasons why good sleep is so important, but other kinds of rest are important too!

## General Recovery

New wearable technology allows you, with some measure of accuracy to track not only your workouts, but your recovery. Being fully recovered prior to a competition, or another serious workout is a great way to be fully alert. Many bad visual habits creep into a player's game when, they are not feeling up to it. Yes, it's true that if you are going to win a 5 hour match, then you will have to train for hours, maintaining great visual discipline and using your skills under tough match conditions. Not fully recovering, can be the reason that you struggle, or even the reason that you give up a slight edge, to an opponent who is fully recovered. The effects are not only physical, but can be mental and emotional, and all three of those things can take a small percentage of acuity away, a percentage that you need, if the match is going to come down to a few shots, at critical times.

## Overtraining

I wanted to explain the very subtle loss of advantage before talking about overtraining, because I didn't want to conflate the two. There are times you are going to significantly challenge your ability to recover, and there are times you must rest. Some commonly understood signs of overtraining, all of them can affect your eyes and your minds interest and ability to follow the ball. If you are in season, and you are responsible to other people like coaches or teammates, let them know what is going on with you, and take a little time to rest up, eat well, and sleep as well as you can.

**Warning Signs**

- Chronic muscle and joint pain
- Weight loss and loss of appetite
- Increased heart rate at rest
- Fatigue
- Prolonged recovery time
- Lack of enthusiasm
- Frequent illnesses
- Difficulty completing usual routines
- Decreased school performance
- Personality or mood changes
- Increased anger or irritability
- Sleep disturbances (difficulty sleeping or sleeping without feeling refreshed)

## Conclusions

Be aware of the issues of environment on your ability to concentrate, and listen to your body about when it's time to push, and/or time to rest. In general, if your workout is so hard that you have a breakdown in concentration or in technique, it's probably good to take a short break, really focus for 5 to 10 minutes, then call it a day. You can expand your capacity by allowing yourself to come back to full concentration and excellent technique for a few minutes while fatigued. However, if you push through while beat, then you will be building in bad visual and stroking habits into your game.

Thirty-Two

## Which Factors Cloud Our Vision? How To Be Alert And Clear Minded On Court.

*Opportunity does not waste time
with those who are unprepared.
~ Idowu Koyenikan*

Our best chance of having great vision is for us to be fully alert. One aspect of Novak Djokovic's dominance at this time on the ATP Tour, is his vision of the ball and the way he prepares to see the ball. If you watch closely you will see that he periodically opens his eyes very wide. This is something I have done myself, and I find that for whatever reason, it seems to reduce the chance of blinking during the return of serve. Blinking affects your vision just enough, that your brain is not able to gather 100% of the visual information, coming from reading the flight of the ball.

**The good news is that our brain is also very good at, filling in some missing information, keeping the world steady in our minds while our eyes our closed for that brief moment.**

Even so, intentionally reducing the regularity of blinking at the worst time, will help us in seeing the ball much better. Since people blink on average 22 times per minute, anxious people blink more often, it stands to reason that calming ourselves, can also reduce the amount of time we have with eyes closed. Speaking of which, a common expression used at Wimbledon in matches with two top servers, 'first one to blink, loses!' I have not found any scientific data to support it, but I believe that great athletes are able to suppress blinking for longer periods of time whether or not they are aware of it. Anything less than 100% visual acuity will introduce some error into the process of tracking and returning the ball, and blinking is the most obvious factor in lost vision.

### Anxiety and Rapid Blinking

Besides anxiety, which other factors may produce a blink? A lack of alertness, early matches, times of natural down time during the day, and fatigue can cause this. Here are a few interventions that can help for these situations:

1. Wake up at least two hours prior to your 8am match, so that you can be

fully awake.

2. Increase your heart rate. If you are heading into a match during a midday lull, snap out of it with some short burst, high intensity exercise, while not compromising your fitness for the match.

3. For a your late match consider taking a nap, or at least a rest with your eyes closed. Resting your eyes for 20 to 45 minutes can refresh your visual acuity from a hard day at work.

4. In the match, rest your eyes briefly between each point, closing your eyes for a moment to visualize can be a two strategy winner. Then let down with the tension in your eyes completely during a changeover. We will get into this more when we talk about the 16 second cure.

## Time Your Blinks, Rest Your Eyes

Obviously, blinking at the time the opponent is making contact, or in the final stages of preparing to make your shot would be the worst times to have your eyes closed. Your eyes need to blink in order to keep them moist, so not blinking for excessively long periods is not advisable, but you can blink at the best time. My guess is that you can blink immediately after you hit your shot, because you will still have time to read the flight of your ball after a microsecond of blinking. This would allow you to blink about every 2 or 3 seconds. I am certain that there are players who fight the need to close their eyes for lengthy periods of time, thus making their eyes tired, and then periodically they close at exactly the wrong time often, and they make errors of because of it. Try to avoid being superhuman. I don't have a conclusive answer, but play around with it and be mindful of your open eye time.

To conclude, I would advise you to experiment with what works for you pay attention to when and how you blink, I'm guessing that if you are a 4.5 player and above, you most likely don't blink at the wrong time often. If you are below that level, perhaps you blink more often, at the wrong time. You can weed out a few errors per set out in your game. Winning three to five more points can make the difference in a close match. So, be alert my friends!

## Fatigue

As a match starts to go deep into third, fourth and fifth sets, depending on the age, experience and conditioning of the players there comes a time where fatigue will set in to your play. As this occurs, it can really play into your ability to concentrate, and thus being fully present with your vision of the ball is at risk. We will address this in a later chapter, but fatigue can definitely disrupt your alertness.

Thirty-Three

## Why Is Eye Protection Controversial?
## Use Different Methods To Protect Your Vision.

*The eye is the lamp of the body, so then if your
eye is clear, your whole body will be full of light.*
~ Jesus

There are no simple answers when it comes to sunglasses, contact lenses, hats, visors or playing in the sun. We can discuss it, and you should think about it intelligently, then take some time to experiment and find what works for you.

### Eye Protection Decisions

Whether to use extra protection of your eyes can be a complex decision. Many players are vehemently opposed to wearing sunglasses, while they play. However, there have been a handful of top 100, even top 10 tennis professionals who always wore them. There are good reasons not to wear sunglasses, and there are many sunglasses that are not at all ideal for sports play. Some sunglasses are actually more harm than help. Wearing hats and visors can help, and there are some other tips for how to deal with the sun that may be helpful in protecting your eyes.

### Sunglasses

Pretty much all sunglasses refract light to some degree, so they will change your normal vision. Some brands claim not to do this, but in reality there will also be some refraction. Even so, search for glassed that have minimal distortion of not only your straight ahead vision, but your peripheral view. Take them on and off, then tilt them to see to what degree they refract light.

Sunglasses also may be too dark and while that is helpful in letting in less light, it may actually be more harmful your eyes than do them any good. Darker sunglasses cause your pupil to increase in size, and that greater opening allows in more radiation to your eye and at angles that are not natural to the natural lighting conditions. Some high level coaches believe that the darker the lens, the harder it is to pick up the ball properly. It seems logical, but I have no hard data to share.

Sunglasses may become steamed up at the wrong time. They can cause you to lose a point. In some conditions the wiping of the sunglasses can become a tiresome, time consuming ritual in between points.

If you wear corrective lenses, it is highly advisable that you gain an expert opinion on whether to have a special pair of sports sunglasses. I use an amber lens at 50% in my prescription sunglasses, and it has made a world of difference to me being able to see more detail in the ball. I am color blind, so that might explain why I am attracted to an amber lens, you might like grey or brown better.

I have worn sunglasses to play for most of my entire adult life, and it took some experimentation to find the best style of lens, color, frame shape, and curvature of lens for my eyes and head.

The next chapter will feature a collection of divergent opinions by coaches at varying levels across the US, and the world, in a question asked in a social media coach's forum.

## Hats and Visors

Putting something on top of your head can work great to keep some of the sun from coming down into your eyes. One thing to look for in a hat or visor is the darkened under-bill of the hat. When the under-bill is black, or another dark color, that helps absorb light that reflects up from the court surface, reducing some glare. In fading afternoon light, you might want a lighter under bill, for exactly the opposite reason.

Some hats and/or visors don't go well with certain sunglasses in the way they fit on your head or over your ears, so that is another thing to consider.

## Sun Vision Skills

We know that direct viewing of the sun is not good for your eyes, but I don't know a tennis player who isn't going try to see a ball in the sun's path. Learning and trying out a few tricks based on the actual location of the sun will give you more strategies for success.

## The Toss

If your normal toss is directly in the sun there are a couple things you can do:

A. Keep your eyes lower and look up at the ball at the latest possible moment.

B. Toss in front of where the sun is, however this will change your serve, you will need a little more lift on your motion.

C. Toss behind the location of the sun, which is less desirable than tossing in front, and you will also need more spin on the shot bring it into the court.

D. Use your tossing hand to partially or fully obscure the sun (without throwing your toss off)

Using the same guidelines you can use the same types of skills on overheads. Don't look up to locate the ball exactly until the last moment, but be sure to track it using peripheral vision. Moving to a place where you can track the ball at an angle that does not include the sun can also be helpful. Good Luck, sometimes it's just plain impossible.  When it's impossible and the ball seems lost in the sun:  HIT THE SUN!

Thirty-Four

## What Are Coach's Opinions On Wearing Sunglasses?

*Your opinion is not my reality.*
*~ Dr. Steve Maraboli*

What are your views, opinions, research on players wearing sunglasses or other eye protection on court? Very few pros have worn sunglasses while playing, why is that?

CC: I think players worry about them falling off or impairing their vision. I feel like I must wear them when I play! I have great vision just can't stand the sun in my eyes and squinting all day on the court. I get headaches.

MH: Avoiding eye damage is a high priority due to constant exposure. I wear them if I'm coaching, playing though I don't see ball as well.

KS: I never wore sunglasses when I competed. I did not see the ball as well with sunglasses on. I do not compete any more. I just play for fun, so it really does not matter.

AS: I play in glasses and have since I discovered I needed them (age 10 or so), so I am used to it and have no issues, but I know others (including my wife) have tried and struggle due to depth perception, so have to wear lenses instead.

SR: Interestingly enough, a large amount of Vitamin D absorption is obtained through the eyes. I wasn't smart enough to have that be my reasoning, but I only wear them when absolutely necessary. Mainly Northward, while serving.

RB: It is similar to wearing a ball cap when playing. You have to do it for a week or two before you become properly accustomed to it. After that it becomes second nature.

ME: I never wore them growing up, but have had eye surgery twice because of sun exposure. Dr. told me he had never had to perform pterygium surgery on someone so young the first time I had it done. Being awake & having someone scrape your eyeball with a scalpel while you lay there, and see it as it's happening was no joke.

CH: To my knowledge (Brand) is the only company that with their lens you don't loose depth perception. I squint so bad in the sun an I can see so much better with the sun glasses on because I can open my eyes all the open. MLB players wear them facing baseball moving in all directions and they still see just fine to hit a 95mph fastball with movement.

DSK: Everyone should wear them, but most don't, as eye damage is real and collective. If you can't do it playing, then do all the other times outside, and while driving. I teach with sunglasses though I believe you would fail the on court with USPTA lesson test with them on, perhaps that has changed. Polarized always, best eyewear is made for mountaineers due to snow reflection.

BF: When I took my USPTA exam 16 years ago (down in Boca Raton, FL), I remember that the written rule was to take the frames off when talking directly to student while not feeding to ensure eye contact. I sometimes forget, but do try to do it to this day.

BC: In my opinion it's absolutely essential to wear state of the art eye wear teaching 95% of lessons. However, when not teaching "foo foo" lessons and you are actually playing or hitting with a VERY high level player, I prefer not using eye wear so I can actually pick up the ball more quickly.

MB: If it doesn't disturb your game go for it! (The Final Word)

Thirty-Five

# How To Use Contact Point Awareness Exercises To Increase Efficiency

*I do not think that word means,
what you think it means.
~ Ynigo Montoya - Princess Bride*

In these next few chapters, there are a wide variety of exercises you can perform, to practice better awareness of different aspects, of the ball's flight and behavior. The secret sauce is in what happens subconsciously, to your reactions and decisions with the ball, as you perform them. The subconcious may be come conscious, and then more deeply subconscious.

**The experimental/experiential practices will engage you to see and experience the ball from a different perspective.**

They can stretch your mind to pay attention to the ball in different ways. Some of these exercises are prescriptions for very specific problems for players need to address. This chapter is largely inspired by the practical suggestions found in *Inner Tennis: Playing the Game*, by W. Timothy Gallway, over time I have worked to develop my own style with each technique.

### Pay Attention to the Contact Point - 'NOW'

Do some rallying, and using 'bounce-hit,' take a little snap shot in your mind of the position of your racquet at contact, at the moment you say, 'hit'. At the moment the ball hits the strings, simply take notice of it's relative position with your arm, in space, with the ball. Don't try to change anything, simply look at how it looks when you make contact.

Take aside some practice time to only really pay attention to the ideal contact point for 5 minutes, and you may see the rest of your practice improve from then onward.

## Top of the Bounce

One game-changing, but fairly subtle adjustment in perception is for a player to see whether the ball is rising or falling. There are funny stories of people telling their experience, but what they say defy the laws of physics. We want to be careful here, because there is no need to fully dispute them, instead understand how they see it. In a conversation with Peter Fadde, Ph.D, who told me a story of a major league baseball player discussing a top pitcher's 'rising' fastball. The problem is that all fastballs go downward.

**The phenomenon of perception stems from the fact that, players have calculated many thousands, if not over a million occurrences, of the average fast ball.**

If a pitcher is able to throw the fastball in a way, that it doesn't fall as much, the batter perceives it as rising compared to the averages of the pitches they normally experience. Is it worth the time and energy to try to convince this player, that there is absolutely no way a fastball could rise? Tennis players will have their own pet ways of experiencing the tennis ball, and we can work with that as long as it works for them. Having said all of that, tennis players will often believe that they have successfully hit the ball on the rise, and coaches will praise them for having done so, or hold unreasonable expectations about how to perform the task. Try using slow motion video to film what is actually happening and the results might surprise you.

**Taking the ball closer to the top of the bounce is perhaps a better way to say it.**

In all my years of coaching, very few players I have seen have intentionally, been able to execute this well, and the best practice seems to be to take the ball just slightly after the incoming shot has peaked and has fallen an inch or two. Of course, there are balls that are hit so well, that the player is under attack, and the only possible way to get a racquet on it is to short hop it, truly taking it on the rise. Roger Federer became legendary, partly due to his ability to take shots from below his knee, driving them deep to corners stunning everyone around the court. He even seemed amazed at times, not really believing that he was the one who hit that stunning winner.

## Film Study

Whether you are player or coach, it's not hard to discover what is really happening. Simply film yourself in a format where playback allows you to watch frame by frame or in slow motion. First, reflect on the most effective 'on the rise' shots that you hit, and then look back on them in video. I believe that you will often see the ball just beginning to fall in those shots.

## Creating An Advantage

Players who take the ball closer to the top of the bounce by choice have a huge advantage over players who fail to take advantage of an opportunity to change the flow of the point. This one factor alone as a determining factor in someone's game can take them up a full level in play and introduce a new weapon in their arsenal.

**The weapon is maximizing their ability to take time away from their opponent.**

I have had quite a few players helped by this process. One girl I coach has all the tools to be a very powerful player, but has been coached previously by those who worship topspin and believe more topspin is always better. Each lesson we seem to spend time straightening this out, but as she improves we spend less and less time on correction and more on very efficient ball striking.

### Marking The Time And Place Verbally

There are two different activities you can try. One is when the ball is incoming, have players say, 'top' when it reaches the highest point between first and second bounce. Then have them attempt to take the ball at the top.

**Even more difficult is to say, 'rising,' 'top,' or 'falling' at the hit, and work very hard to take the ball while rising.**

This is when you can check the relative differences in perception, of the contact with the ball. What I also think you will find is that when players truly do take the ball on the rise, the results will not be satisfactory. Learning the difficult shot, of taking the ball at the top, is made a bit more difficult when a player is fooled into thinking, that they are taking it on the rise, while they are not really doing it.

Thirty-Six

# Can We Improve Our Focus?
# How To Improve Ability
# To Focus Without Saccads.

*Your eyes are a muscle, and they need
training like all your muscles.
~ Visian ICL*

While evidence from 2015 suggests that we ought not to try to maintain perfect focus, or pinpoint vision, of the ball during its entire flight, a great overtraining exercise can prepare you to maximize your ability focus on the ball for longer periods of time. All of the exercises below will help you overcome eye fatigue, computer vision syndrome, and help with various aspects of eye performance, including being able to focus in the best way for longer.

## Your Fingerprint and The Cyclone Fence

Stand at the baseline. Raise your index finger up. With your finger print about 8 to 12 inches from your face, focus on your fingerprint until you can see it perfectly. Take notice of how everything in the background will be blurry, and you will have double vision of most objects. From your fingerprint, shift your focus to the far fence, pick a small object on the fence on which to focus, preferably at the same height which you would be looking at a server's toss.

Did you feel your focus shifting away from the focus point on your finger to the fence? Now shift it back, did you feel it shifting back to your finger?

Slowly shift again and again, then shift it more quickly but smoothly from your finger back to the fence 4 times. Do one more repetition of 4, that should be enough for that exercise.

This will exercise your eyes to smoothly shift focus. I have heard it said that your vision can shift at upwards of 120 MPH, but I have no data. If it's wrong, its not wrong by much.

## Maximum Speed and Practical Application

Once you begin to feel very comfortable, then experiment with focusing on the far fence all the way to your fingerprint and have your focus shift as fast as possible, as though you were following a ball in flight. Now do this faster and faster.

Now go and rally some tennis balls and try to maintain focus on the ball during an entire rally. Of course, when you are tracking you can work to keep the ball fairly close to the center of your vision. It's obvious that this is contradictory to other advice in this book, but we have already established that the visual system is somewhat mysterious, so I remain open minded to any intervention that might work for any particular player. It has proven though, that trying to focus on an object moving directly across your vision, while trying to have pinpoint accuracy will lead to saccadic motion of the eye and losing sight of the ball, so practice this, with that in mind.

## Three Stage Eye Training

Start with your finger one foot from your face, maintain focus for 15 full seconds, while moving your finger to arms length away. Now find something in the distance at least 15 feet away and focus on that for 15 seconds. You will see that focusing more for than a few seconds is actually not very easy.

## Figure 8

Look at a relatively uniform area without much detail like a floor or undecorated wall. Move your eyes in a figure 8, same motion as an infinity symbol, do this five times in each direction. You will find it difficult at first, but then the motion of your eyes will become more smooth as the muscles of your eyes learn to work together more efficiently.

## Doing Eye Rolls

Take your eyes around in full circles 3 times in each direction.

## Looking to 8 Directions

Move your eyes in each direction as far as you comfortably can. There is a science that believes that looking in different directions engages different parts of your brain. Body language experts look to see if people are looking in one direction to access real memories, and another direction to access creative modalities.

Thirty-Seven

## Does Everyone Process Visually At The Same Speed?  Understanding Factors That Effect Visual Processing

*One type of processing speed is visual processing speed, this is the most common kind referred to. Visual processing speed is how fast your child can look at and process information on a task that does not take any more thinking than noticing the differences or sameness in the objects shown. This type of processing speed issue may be helped by vision therapy, or larger print. Extra time on tests is important so the child has time to correctly "see" the information and not make careless errors due to misreading the information. When children also have difficulty with fine motor skills (writing) this becomes a visual-motor integration weakness. Another type of processing speed is cognitive processing speed. This is how long it takes a child to process (take in information, think about it and then give an answer). This type of child also needs extra time on tests, not "see" the information but to "think" about the answer.*
*~ Melissa Mullen, Ph.D.*

Everyone has some type of processing delay.  Consider this, someone said something to you, then later when thinking about it, you understand what they meant.  Or you are taking a class, are confused, and then in your next class you have an 'a-ha' moment from the previous class' instruction.  That's a great example of how processing works. Very often I will have had a fairly lengthy break from teaching a student, due to bad weather, illness, business or whatever.  When they come back, they are better, and they learned the skill that they were struggling with in the prior lesson, but with no further practice or teaching.

**Their brain was still busy learning.**

Even during the off time, that allowed more processing of experiences. In discussion of particular types of processing delays that happen in the moment, there is no shame in having a longer arc of processing in a particular skill.  It's important to understand how you differ from others in processing, but also do what you can to improve your capacity. If you are a coach you want to discover this in the player's you coach. You also want to discover the relative strengths in how you think, compared with those around you.

## People Have Their 'Go To' Mode

A player's favored learning modality can play a huge factor, in how they see a ball, in a training situation or live play. From my experience as a high school algebra teacher, I learned that some students have delayed verbal processing skills, and others have delayed visual processing. As I began to experiment with this, in the classroom, I found that there are students who were working very hard to overcome their relatively slow verbal processing speed. Because they were trying so hard to hear and understand the words I was saying, and this ran right into their weakness, it consumed much of their brains CPU. With all that bandwidth taken up by listening, their eyes had a diminished ability to see. In their effort to overcome their deficit in verbal processing, they then could not see as well, unable to process quickly what was happening, as I showed examples of solving problems on the whiteboard.

**One day, I decided to teach without talking for as long as I possibly could, or while using the absolute fewest words possible.**

I very slowly solved an algebra equation math, that multiple students had missed on a recent homework assignment, showing the steps repeatedly. In demonstrating how to solve the problem, I also showed the steps of my work, then erased them. This made some of the stronger verbal processing students angry that I wasn't talking, which fed into their strength. I had to shush them from protesting, "Why aren't you talking!". Suddenly, one student erupted with "NOW I GET IT!" When I asked them why they got it, they stated that since they didn't have to listen, then they could see what I was doing, fresh for the first time. You can try the same thing with your students, holding a relatively silent lesson. If you are a player, you will be best advised to have minimal talking in training sessions, of course some talking will be necessary. Tennis is not math class, and our work in learning the game is very heavily in the arena of seeing and feeling, the visual and the kinesthetic awareness of what we are doing. It's far better to train our brains in that awareness, then to stay in our 'go to' verbal processing.

## Visual Processing Compromised

The people at Billie Jean King's Eye Coach recently conducted an in depth study on vision, and found that multitasking while learning tennis is not the best method. Since that time, I have dramatically reduced and simplified anything I might say, while there are live balls in play. In between points, I might make a quick comment to a player, then give them a few seconds to process the information, before checking understanding. Players may then be better prompted, to see what we want them to see, when we give them a separate moment, to hear what it is. This will no doubt continue, to be of some frustration, to those who are the faster verbal processors.

**They can learn to be patient and operate out of a different modality as well.**

I occasionally lose a student, because they are so hell bent on having me offer complicated explanations of the process of hitting a tennis ball. The attending tension they exhibit in trying to perform all of those nuances with a 'checklist' in their mind, informs me not to teach that way. When they insist, and I push back by explaining that it takes them away from simple awareness of what they are doing, their reaction will tell if we are going to be working together much longer. As a student myself, and I'm guessing that many of you have had the same experience, I was sometimes frustrated by those in a class who seemed to always raise their hand first. I found myself raising my hand, as though to win some kind or race, even though I had not thought out my answer. Since that time, I have learned to slow myself down to process at a slower speed, for greater accuracy in listening. Conversely, I work hard to reduce reaction time, and increase the efficiency of decision making skills in my players. People with faster answers are not necessarily more intelligent than those with verbal processing delay. It's not a race to the first answer, it's about taking a little time to process the best answer.

### 'Think' Time

In teaching credential programs, teachers learn about 'think time'. It's a great idea to give yourself and others time to think. It's easy to be impatient, not wanting any silence. When I ask children questions at the end of a lesson with their parents present, it's strange to see the parent urging their child on to answer, before they have even had a few seconds to think. I don't demand answers from my players, often. Sometimes I get a lazy thinker, who answers a question with a question. I ask them "Why did you miss that shot?" and then they immediately shoot back with "Why?", so then I let them know that I am asking them the question, so they can answer why they missed the shot. I have a little girl who when she was 6, not knowing the answer was quite upsetting to her, but now that she is 8, she understands what lead to a missed shot, she can reflect back on her performance and see that her spacing to the ball was too close.

It's fairly easy to recognize the strong verbal processing players, because they are almost always the first to answer a question. Of course, in their haste, they may answer incorrect. Wrong answers are ok, because they allow the coach to understand that the player does not understand. Partially correct answers give you a moment to affirm what is right, but then also redirect what was not correct. When receiving or giving coaching, allow yourself and others time to compare what is being said with what is seen and felt. At the end of every lesson, I want to hear what my players saw or felt during the lesson, because their experience of it is far more important than their thoughts, analysis, check list or any other verbal form of organizing the information. Every lesson you take, try to come away with one, two or three takeaways that are visual, kinesthetic, or kinematic.

To conclude, consider the duration and timing spoken communication in how you are learning or teaching the game. A best practice is to use words that are analogous to what really happens on a tennis court. For example, "It's like throwing the tip of the racquet at the ball" for a serve. There are endless examples, and I like to understand my student's other sports experiences, to draw comparisons to things they do in baseball, basketball, etc. The words you use can best express 'feel-mages' according to Tim Gallwey. Words work best when they paint a picture or explain how something feels. The final thought is that it's great to try to use fewer words, while demonstrating what you want to be seen and imitated, and engage feeling by shadow swinging or guiding the racquet in exactly the path you want it to go to gain the feeling. The more you can create an image to imitate, and guide the feeling that the player can experience the better. Those are part of the old school wisdom of learning the game.

Thirty-Eight

## Why Move Away From Pinpoint Vision And Toward 'Bounce-Hit'?

*Life is one big road with lots of signs. So when you riding through the ruts, don't complicate your mind. Flee from hate, mischief and jealousy. Don't bury your thoughts, put your vision to reality. Wake Up and Live!*
*~ Bob Marley*

As discussed in the introduction, the inspiration for this book came from watching a documentary about the football catching skills of Steve Largent. Steve is perhaps the greatest possession style wide receiver in NFL history and his ability to catch in traffic, and while laid completely out in a full diving motion is legendary. Steve said that while most people tried to focus on the ball, he tried to focus on the tiny X that is formed in the stitching on the forward point of the ball. He claims that this helped him more than anything to get in the right position for the catch.

**This, of course, is supported by the research which shows that the angle of focus is approximately 3 degrees in front of us**.

Focusing on a smaller part of the ball, helps keep the ball in focus, for a longer period of time. Explaining when and where that focus happens, and how much of it was in Steve's imagination is something we can't discuss. What he experienced, and what he truly strove for in his visual skill, may be very close to 100% peculiar to him, and not advisable for many people to attempt. One thing that makes a wide receiver's job more difficult and unlike a tennis player is that they will not often see the ball coming out of the hand of the QB, so having a smaller anchor point for vision to pick up the ball mid-flight is quite helpful.

### Experiencing the Ball

On a tennis court, reading and reacting to a tennis ball is perhaps more critical, because we don't have a quarterback who is throwing the ball to us, but an opponent who is keeping the ball away from us, and to the most inconvenient place they can.

There are quite a few different exercises and drills we can practice to gain better detail in our experience of the flights of a tennis ball. Simply attempting to gain greater detail, can give better results. W. Tim Gallway in *Inner Tennis: Playing the Game*, the second book in the Inner Game of Tennis franchise, fleshes out in greater detail a very strong menu of visual cue drills which are very practical, even if they are not always easily understood.

## Bounce-Hit

This is a very simple awareness exercise which brings your mind's attention only to what you can see. Start by saying 'bounce' when the ball bounces, and say 'hit' when the ball makes contact with your strings. This drill demands that you pay attention to the exact time that the ball bounces and the exact time that you are hitting the ball. Try to say those words exactly when they happen. Players discover that they might not have been seeing the ball accurately, that anxiety causes them to think the ball is traveling faster than it is, or that they have hit the ball earlier than they thought they would.

This exercise could be your most ideal place to start with visual training, as it helps solve problems where the problem of perception lies, at the ball bounce and contact point.

Players often report that they felt like the ball had slowed down, but in reality, they had slowed their perception of the ball down to a slower speed. Using this method naturally brings interest and full attention to two critical moments to the ball bounce and contact with the strings, instead of commanding it. The timing of 'hit' is mainly a kinesthetic exercise because you can't really see the ball hit the strings, but you can feel it. The pairing of the visual and the kinesthetic is part of the magic of 'bounce-hit'. This also leads to a light hypnotic trance, and thus relaxed concentration. n

## NOT 100% Effective

Over 25 years of using this exercise, I would say it works for 85% to 90% of my students, and for some, it just does not work at all. A small group of people really hate doing it. My personal theory is that those who have an issue of delayed processing in speech, are the ones that are most distracted by trying to form the words, and their attention goes away from the ball. For those players, I may have them make a noise, like clicking their tongue, or blowing a little air out of the mouth.

After a period of time where my student has begun to master this, and their timing has improved dramatically, then I ask them to use 'bounce-hit' on both sides of the court, their side and my side. This completes the exercise, as it sums up the understanding of the whole system of hitting a ball, following its course to the opponent's strings, seeing their hit, tracking and reacting to its new course, fine tuning footwork and arriving at the ideal place for a great shot. Bottom line: If you seem to be someone who doesn't like this exercise, there is nothing wrong with you, and there are other great things you can do.

## Internalizing For Unconscious Competence

Doing bounce hit, or even saying bounce, followed by the number of the rally is a conscious competence exercise. After a period of time of saying it out loud, which is important to do until you are fairly accurate about saying it on time, then you can begin to say it very softly, and finally say it in your mind internally for a few minutes before letting it fade away. Ultimately the internalizing of the skill is the most important, because you can't say bounce hit out loud in your match. Maybe you can move your lips and make the sound barely audible to anyone on court, but it's far better to keep it internal while playing. Once you get to that level, you have achieved an unconscious competence.

Some say good players don't have time to say 'bounce-hit' but, I don't agree. Even if that were true, you can easy substitute a tongue click, or an exhale or light grunt as a timing mechanism. I would never advocate loud grunting. In the next chapter, we will go over even more detailed methods for tracking the ball.

*Whenever I find myself out of rhythm or concentration, I return to 'bounce-hit'!*

Thirty-Nine

## Do We Have It Backwards? Challenge The Visual System With Overtraining, Before Introducing A Larger Ball

*For any fitness component to improve, it must be overloaded. To obtain optimal improvement and prevent injury, overload must be individualized and progressive.*
*~ (Hodge, Sleivert, McKenzie 1996)*

The Overtraining Principle should not be confused with Overtraining Syndrome. The Principle is about engaging in activities that are more difficult than the actual task you will need to perform. The syndrome is a collection of symptoms that indicate an athlete is training too much, too often, or without enough recovery. It's not a stretch to use the overload, overtraining principle for your eyes.

**My players regularly train their eyes with tasks more difficult than actual play.**

When you do this, you create a comparison that the competition is actually easy and fun. Two legendary basketball coaches, Pete Newell and John Wooden, were well noted for running practices that were so difficult that the games seemed easier in comparison. Of course, they also made sure that their players were rested for the game.

**Caution: Using Golf Balls is Dangerous. Do Not Attempt.**

In my crazier days, I have had my players play with golf balls. Yes, they hit golf balls with tennis rackets. It didn't take long to find out how dangerous the golf ball drill really is, so only my very best and most disciplined players were allowed to participate in the challenge. It was important to reinforce to them, that they would need to take very short backswings for the ball.

Not only is a golf ball more difficult to track due to its size and color, but the impact on the strings is more dramatic, due to the interaction with the hard and uneven surface created by dimples on the ball.

After only a few short rallies with golf balls, for a maximum of about 10 minutes we saw a dramatic increase in a player's vision of a tennis ball. All the players were amazed that, in comparison, the tennis ball seemed to look like a grapefruit and seemed to be traveling so slowly.

We have also tried rubber 'super' balls, but the way those balls interact with the court surface picking up spin might make them even more dangerous, and less realistic in their bounce, since they are even more lively than a golf ball.

### Smaller Objects

Finally, there is one product that is much safer to play with, and about 80% as effective in overtraining the eye, without the risk of injury or court damage. There is a promotional product for tennis that works fairly well. I now use a foam stress ball tennis ball keychain. I remove the keychain mechanism from the stress ball and rally with it with my students. The best thing about this is, that students of all ages can safely use it. The problem is that teenagers find that they can hit the ball right at the coach, and that it doesn't hurt as much as a tennis ball, so they are tempted to continue trying to hit the coach, instead of focusing on the drill at hand.

**I use this approximately 1.5" diameter ball mainly for volleys, but if you play up close, and are O.K. with two bounces sometimes, it can be used for groundstrokes.**

This has the opposite effect from using red balls, which are larger. I find that using smaller balls with smaller children is far more beneficial visually, although the red balls bouncing slower and lower for youngsters seems to be also a great advantage in their training, so be sure to do both. Confidence found in the success of the shots is the ultimate goal, but the long term training of the to do more difficult things is the hidden process.

In addition, there is no real data, but in my discussions with many great tennis coaches, there is a strong sentiment that junior players who train with Red, Orange, Green Dot AND YELLOW BALLS, outperform those who only train with the colored compression balls. Of course, if you add even smaller balls to the training, along with stationary ball training and, other ways to train vision as found in this book and you will have the completely trained player. These different experiences will also help players to learn to detect the subtle differences in how the ball behaves in different conditions: Dry, High Altitude, Cold, Extreme Heat, Heavy Damp, etc.

**Be sure to keep it safe!**

Forty

## What Is The Sequence To Check For Visual Errors? Know The Five F's Of The Visual System

*Man is not born to solve the problem of the universe,
but to find out what he has to do; and to restrain
himself within the limits of his comprehension.*
~ *Johann Wolfgang von Goethe*

When you want to diagnose where a breakdown occurs in the visual system, we always start from the beginning, like a mechanic that first checks the battery of a car that won't start. If we look at the very simple system of a ball traveling back and forth between two players, then we can detect where the initial breakdown in visual skills occurred.

### The System Is An Interaction Between Players

These things flow one into another, but you can start to discover if you have a problem in any segment.:
1. The opponent makes contact. Do you pay full attention to that moment?

2. Once the ball is out of the frame by 2 feet, your brain with 95% accuracy knows where it is going. Do you begin moving immediately? This is a place of considerable training and habit forming.

3. The ball is a blur and flies over the net to the bounce. Are you tracking it, trusting your brains ability to get it into your strings?

4. The ball bounces and slows down dramatically. Prior to the bounce, are you relatively still and focusing either on the ball, or a place halfway between the bounce and contact? (Of course, some very well hit shots by the opponent will have you scrambling)

5. You make contact through to follow through. Is your head relatively still during the entire swing? Are you on balance? Is the ball well placed in the strings?

6. You have finished your swing. Did you turn your gaze to see where your

ball bounced, then to the opponent to see the ball come out of their strings?

With a nod to Oscar Wegner, I want to share my 5 F's of visual awareness, largely influenced by that great coach and his 'Find, Feel, Finish'.

## Find The Ball

When the ball strikes the opponent's racquet, find the ball coming out as quickly as possible. Of the many words available for seeing something, 'find' is one that has a connotation of taking interest in it. Finding an object sounds a lot more interesting, than focusing on it. One word sounds likes discovery, the other like work. Even though 'scan' might be a more accurate technical term for the function your eyes perform, 'find' may seem more user friendly.

In the art of teaching visual skills, finding the ball may fit better with the human system, than other terms, that might make better sense, as part of a clinical study.

As mentioned previously, one of my 2021 discoveries is the importance of the word 'where' and why knowing where the ball is, where you want to meet it, and where you want to hit it. 'Where' flows through the faster pathways of your brain. Recent neuroscience is showing, that disengaging the frontal cortex, while in the act of playing allows for better flow state. Finding the ball does that.

Finding, also seems to mesh well with Vic Braden's assertion about our brain's ability to extrapolate the landing place of the ball with great accuracy, when we attend to the immediate beginning of its flight. Quite commonly in working with my players, the source of early errors in a lesson, clinic, or match are not attending to finding the ball out of the opponent's strings.

## Footwork to the Ball

'Find' and 'Footwork' are so closely connected, that top players make their initial move to a ball much more quickly, than those below them in the rankings and they are very difficult to fool with a shot. In Novak Djokovic's groundbreaking performance in the final of the 2019 Australian open, the nearly instantaneous first step in the split second after Nadal's contact, was the most important determining factor for the domination.

I tell my players that there is 'on time' preparation and there is 'late preparation,' but there is no such thing as 'early'. Training the most efficient reaction to the ball is critical for top flight play. The lag time between finding the ball and the initiation of footwork, is a dividing factor among players of different levels. When players aspire to a new level, initially the speed of the ball will be a challenge to which they must adapt, through improved reactions to what they see. This is where the direct connection of the Ocular Nerve to muscle nerve tissue comes into play. Getting to the unconscious competence necessary to instantly react, is key to this automatic instinctual play.

The most important issue here, is to train increasingly more efficient reactions, so as to aid in instinctual reactions of the unconsciously competent player at work. Most all of learning includes moving from, not knowing that you don't know something, this ignorance is called 'Unconscious Incompetence'. The instructor may ask a question that we don't know the answer to, and that points out 'Conscious Incompetence,' when you now know that there is something you didn't previously know. When you learn something for the first time, especially when it runs counter to a habitual pattern to which you are accustomed, then you need 'Conscious Competence' to think your way through it, but too many players live in that zone, failing to move into 'Unconscious Competence' where you have practiced something well enough that you do it automatically. You can very quickly learn to trust yourself, in making a first move to a ball!

## Feel the Ball

As noted previously, 90% of mishits are the result of poor vision of the ball. Using mishits as a barometer for feedback about effectiveness of vision, we can then assume that either: the vision of the ball was off, or the accuracy of the footwork was not precise. From experience with players of many levels, I find that the vast majority are able to recognize poor positioning, although some find it difficult to know if they were too close, or too far away from the ball. Then comes the myriad ways to move to balls that are further, closer, coming at your body.

**The training of the full lexicon of movement patterns, that may take some years to master is a step by step, 'cross that bridge when you get it' endeavor.**

Players are wise to discover which kind of shot gives them the most trouble, first learning to recognize when that shot is coming, to which part of the court. 'Ball Recognition' was a passing fad in tennis coaching a few years back, but I don't remember anyone discussing visual skills, as they pertain to the concept. Recognition presumes that someone, has seen a particular kind of shot before, and has some experience in attempting to hit it back, good or bad. In reality, how you use your eyes to identify the flight of the incoming ball, is the most essential piece of the puzzle to reacting properly, so that you can position yourself to feel the ball in the best part of your racquet.

### After the Follow Through

As you continue to follow through, shortly thereafter, you must begin to read the flight of your own ball, as it travels to your opponent. People make the mistake of being so outcome focused, and evaluative, with their shot, even stooping to subjective judgements about whether their shot was good or bad, that they fail to actually finish their shot, thus increasing the chances of a less effective shot.

**Wait until after you have finished your follow through, at least, to begin looking for the landing spot of your shot.**

With experience, many predictive cues come into play, as you see the effect of your shot on the opponent, and begin to see their move to the ball, which will help you to calculate a range of possible shots on their end. Depending on how good your shot is, you might have left the opponent with their only smart shot being a lob, but that doesn't mean they might not try for a desperate winner and make it. If you hit the ball in the center of the court and bouncing up nicely, you can expect an offensive shot from the other player who has had any training in taking those offensively.

## Finish the Stroke

When exactly should a player pick up visually, the flight of their outgoing ball? Sometime after they have completed their follow through, and around the time their own ball crosses the net. Styrling Strother's notion of 'Ball/Player' is a strong one, in that it's more important to take note of your opponent and what your ball is doing to them, rather than simply become fascinated with your own shot. You will then begin to pick up visual cues in your opponent's game.

Immediately after you 'finish,' in the recovery or relaxation stage of your stroke, the recognition of the outcome of your shot, will allow you to discover where to move to in the court, to prepare for the next shot. In this phase it's very helpful to allow yourself to get a full relaxation phase in your shot, although if the other player's shot was very stressful, at your feet, or putting you on the dead run, you most likely won't have that luxury. There are so many contingencies, and that's why tennis is such a great sport.

Many players begin running for the next shot prior to finishing their last shot. Beginning to move for your next shot, before completing the one you are hitting, compromises your efficiency, and is mostly born out of anxiety. Players begin to rush when they have the feeling, as if there is not enough time to prepare.

**They then lose a bit of efficiency, and the quality of your shot is diminished.**

Not finishing a stroke properly can allow for a better chance for your opponent will have a higher quality opportunity to play a better shot back to you. Learning to stay in the shot until its completion, THEN recovering will lead to better overall results. Remember that the opponent can't hit the ball until after you do, and it does take time for your ball to get to them, they can't hit it until it arrives.

Each point is a process that repeats from finding the ball, positioning ourselves to feel the ball, using a proper finish, sighting the outgoing ball, then the whole process repeats.

Forty-One

## Stop Saying "Watch The Ball" And Learn To Give Full Attention To The Ball

*I'm so poor, I can't afford to pay attention.*
*~ Jack Baugh*

### at·ten·tion (ə-těn′shən) n.

1.a. The act of close or careful observing or listening: You'll learn more if you pay attention in class.

b. The ability or power to keep the mind on something; the ability to concentrate: We turned our attention to the poem's last stanza.

c. Notice or observation: The billboard caught our attention.

The primary definition of attention has subtle variations that can help us give more ability to be fully present. The root of the word is attend, and the original latin is a verb — 'to stretch'. Attending has connotations of being present, and the middle English definition is to 'use your mental faculties', according to google this word has declined in usage over the years.

Yes, we need to carefully observe the flight of the ball, and the sound of the ball also paired with the sight give an indication of how well the ball has been struck.

Advanced tennis players have stretched their ability to concentrate, for long periods of time, well above the norm. Being fully present, not distracted on court is not easy. The fact that you will lose 45-49% of the points in a match that you will easily win, means almost every other point you have an opportunity to get distracted. But, giving our full attention to the ball, while also accounting for our opponent's court position demands that we move away from distraction, attend to the matters of relaxation, planning, ritual to be fully prepared for the next point coming, while having noted important information from the point prior.

### Love the Ball

Billie Jean King was noted for having a ritual where she would place a ball in front of her and say repeatedly, 'I love the ball'. Bringing an emotional attachment to the object can help make the experience complete, probably more so for some people, than others. While I forget the reference, someone important quoted or coined the phrase, 'only the ball' as a mantra to be repeated between points. The ball is really the only thing that matters, as you don't play the opponent, you play the ball they hit.

Consider the different aspects of attention, and see how it's multifaceted, and perhaps we come to an understanding that attention is greater than the sum of its parts. Tennis pulls our attention outside of ourselves to an amazing challenge of better awareness of a fuzzy yellow object, that can be quite captivating and two balls never come the same way.

**Multi-Tasking**

I have certain players who do a lot of multitasking in their minds. When I see a distracted player, we stop what we are doing for a moment, to ask, "How many different things do you have going on in your head right now", the answer is sometimes two, three, or even five or more. I ask the player to then take a moment and tell those other thoughts that are not the ball to go away until after court time is over. Those thoughts create distractions for paying full attention to the ball. It's quite possible that, those thoughts will pop back up, but gently you can tell them to stop. One great strategy to help with this is to say, 'stop', and in that moment you have an opening, and then the next thing you should say is, 'only the ball'. If any other comes back, tell it what time you are going to think about it again. Yes, talk to it, but not outloud, for obvious reasons. You do need those thoughts, but not at this time in your match or practices. You may be surprised how little practice it takes to learn to turn off thoughts that are not working for you at the moment.

Forty-Two

# On Court Visual Challenge Drills
# (Part One)
# Live Ball Play and Ball Machines

*Progress is man's ability to complicate simplicity.*
*~ Thor Heyerdahl*

Each of these on court drills will challenge different capacities of visual ability, from the ability to shift attention from one object to another, creating opportunities to see the court differently, maintain awareness of one object and take the ability to track fast moving objects to the maximum.

## Rally Two Balls at Once

One of the classic drills to challenge your visual system, is to rally two balls with a partner. It's a classic overtraining exercise. For a moment, your full attention must go to the ball you are about to hit, but then you will immediately shift your attention to the next incoming ball. Let me ask you two questions, that I can't answer at the moment.

**Will this drill deprive your ability to see the ball coming out of the opponent's racquet, or improve your ability to be aware of it in your peripheral vision?**

Will the drill require you to pay better attention to your contact point, trusting your ability to track the incoming yellow blur? Try both methods. Either way, when you get done with this drill, the requirement of hitting only one ball will seem like a relative luxury.

Start at the T for short court, and focus on hitting with equal rhythm and speed with your partner. The longer you can maintain a rally where you each are hitting around the same time makes it easier, if the balls start to come too fast, hit the second one higher and slower to increase the amount of time between shots. This is a great thing to do for around 5 - 10 minutes, although you could turn it into a game where you rally the two balls, then when one ball goes out, then the second ball is live for a point. A variation of this is called Dingles, where 4 people rally two balls, and when one ball is missed, then the second ball becomes live and counts for the point. It teaches outside awareness beyond what you are currently doing.

### Team Singles

This drill is actually not very challenging for an individual, but it opens up new understanding, and works great with intermediate players to develop better court awareness. 3 to 6 players can play this, more than 6 makes it a slow game. Play rally points, and each player must alternate shots. So if you have players A, B, and C, then A must hit the first ball, followed by B and so on...

**If a player fails to hit a shot, then they will get the next ball in the next point.**

With three players only, one of them will play alone, while the other two will alternate shots, play one game to 7 or 11, then rotate so that everyone gets two chances to play team singles, and one chance to play alone. The effect is that players wait to see the outcome of the player ahead of them, then that shot coming from the opponent. They start to have awareness of what the opponent is actually doing, because they are standing relatively still and not engaged yet in the point. This creates a bridge to being able to perform the same skill while engaged in a point.

### Short Court Chaos

Cross court short court, with 4 players and balls crossing back and forth is also a good thing to do. If you have 6 players, you can put two players outside the court diagonally opposite of each other making extreme angles working to get the ball in the alley opposite of them on the other side of the court. Then, four players can have cross court short court rallies, and now you have balls going every which way you can.

**There is also a good chance balls will collide in mid air, that is one fun element of the game.**

If coaching a large group, give a reward for players who can make balls collide in midair. Pro-Tip: have players feed the first shot almost simultaneously, so that their feed has a secondary target of another ball in the air, while also trying to hit the primary target on the other side.

### Ball Machine - Progressively Faster

With any number of people, you can use a ball machine to very slowly increase the speed or spin of shots, and make a game of how many errors they can make. If you want the game to go faster, eliminate people after 2 errors, and if you want it to go longer then use 5 errors. Depending on what your ball machine can do, you might also make greater distances between shots, and eventually go all the way to the maximum speed of what it will make in the court, with no spin for maximum challenge. This turns a scary situation into a fun challenge, and you can reverse the anxiety by taking a challenge approach, because no one is expected to be perfect in this situation. You can also find out who is challenged at lower speeds, and at increasing speeds. Of course, your best players are more likely to survive to the end, but you might be surprised.

## Practicing With Only One Ball

I find that my students make 50% fewer errors, and also learn more from each one when they or I have to go get the ball when it gets away. It gives space to think, to feed the imagination, to give both of us time to reflect. A basket of 375 balls gives 374 excuses to miss. One ball is unforgiving, and when it's gone, you have none. One ball is all that is ever in play in a match, so you must take care of it just the same.

Forty-Three

## On Court Visual Challenge Drills
## (Part Two)
## Contact Point, Pairing The Swing

*Sometimes I've believed as many as six
impossible things before breakfast.
~ Lewis Carroll*

### Seeing the Top of the Ball

This might not seem like a contact point exercise, but let me explain....As the ball gets closer, it will begin to take up more than 3 degrees of your vision, so picking a smaller part of the ball to see gives more precise vision with the *Steve Largent Effect*. Start with looking at the top of the ball, this will help certain players. Some players find it quite difficult to hit anything but topspin, many times they hit too much topspin, to the point where their balls lack power, landing short in the court.

These players may try very hard to learn to flatten out the ball in practice, but when live ball play resumes, they go back to hitting more topspin than is helpful, necessary, or appropriate.

The problem seems to be, that they perceive the ball as being lower than it really is. So, they prepare their racquet lower to the ball, than they should. Then, they are perpetually surprised by the ball arriving higher, than they thought, thus brushing way up to it. It's amazing to me how this is missed, by players and coaches, and even encouraged wrongly.

For a reason I can't explain, players actively looking at the top of the ball, seem to more accurately judge it's true height, and are able to prepare the racquet, at a corresponding height. Almost immediately upon taking notice of the top of the ball, the player learns to raise the racquet, to an appropriate height for more of a topspin drive shot.

Of course, there may need to be some modeling of taking the racquet back a little higher, and/or not allowing the racquet to drop too low below the contact point.

After minimal intervention, pairing the better perception, with better execution, can happen very quickly, even though it may take a bit longer, for the new habit to take shape. From that moment it's just a matter of mindful practice, keeping an eye at the top of the ball, and developing greater racquet awareness.

## Seeing the Bottom of the Ball

Paying close attention to the bottom of the ball has the opposite effect, assisting players who need to slice, or better yet, hit some topspin instead of only hitting flatter shots. With the same rationale as stated above, some players struggle to hit topspin, and may only hit flatter shots (yes it's true that about 1 in 10,000 shots actually has zero spin). These same players may regularly slice balls that would be best addressed with topspin.

If the player tunes into the bottom of the ball, they almost magically adjust, making the transition to getting their racquet lower, underneath the ball, so that they can come up behind it.

They can learn to keep their racquet lower below the ball, to produce the topspin that they need, to keep the ball in play, or make angled shots on court. It's the same principle, as top of the ball, in reverse. It's not my intention to start a conversation about ideal technique about how to hit ideal topspin, instead I recommend that you and your players learn to hit a variety of spins from a topspin drive, a high looping ball, a short angle, a low 'dip-drive,' the 'buggy-whip,' and a topspin lob in order to be a complete player.

## Use Slow Motion

To understand visual best technique, the use of slow motion video is one of the greatest advancements learning to play tennis. This helps players to see what they could not see, and thus develops their imagination, giving them a framework to reconcile the result of scans, tracks, and foci. An incredible amount of additional information can be gained, that the unaided human eye could not previously detect.

As a result of using slo-motion video, I now have almost no disagreements with players about what they are doing with their stroke, since they can see it very easily.

Not only can they see their stroke, but they can also compare it to their experience of the ball in real time, thus gaining a much better understanding of how to translate their perception into more efficient action. We can trace the very origin of the maladaptive motion.

## Pair Visual and Kinesthetic with Video

The connection that you can make with images, can have a dramatic and relatively permanent positive effect, on your game in the pairing of the tracking of the ball, with getting into an ideal position in which to receive it in your strings. An ideally positioned point of contact will aid you in getting relatively on balance, with good posture, and with the ball in an ideal spot in your strings.

**Contrary to conventional wisdom, the sweet spot is not always the ideal place to strike the ball, but that is the subject of an advanced tennis lesson.**

Good posture actually allows you to lean ever so slightly onto the contact point, so it's not perfectly straight up ballerina posture that is ideal. You can tell how well you were balanced for your shot, based on whether you have to lean, or step immediately, after your shot. When you can simply remain in place, coming to completely balanced ready position after your shot, then you were in ideal position for it.

Slow motion video removes any denial about what is happening, making for a much more powerful lesson. You can begin to detect the smaller amounts of inaccurate movement, training your eyes move excellently to get you in position. Players can then also pair the visual, with the kinesthetic experience, and can be more ready to make a change, once they are aware what exactly they are doing. Vision is clearly a major component to learning how to be a great player.

**Quite often I ask my players, "Do you see and/or feel what you did there? Which one had the greater impact, the seeing or the feeling?"**

This helps me to tap into which is their stronger modality. Of course, all of us tennis players see and feel, and pairing these two makes our learning very powerful. This jibes with Tim Gallwey's idea of 'feel-mages', expressed in The Inner Game of Tennis, as the way to learn how to repeatedly perform a certain task. So, get creative with different ways of having your players experience their shots.

Forty-Four

# On Court Visual Challenge Drills
# (Part Three)
# Ball Flight Awareness

*The best way to capture moments is to pay attention.*
*This is how we cultivate mindfulness.*
*Mindfulness means being awake.*
*It means knowing what you are doing.*
*~ on Kabat-Zinn*

## Satellite in Space

Just like the moon has its different phases, based on its position in relation to the sun and earth, the ball has a lighter side and darker side which changes as it 'orbits' the court. When following the ball, try to see the shaded part of the ball for a few shots, then track the light side. Take note of the different experience you might have on an overcast day, or when the sun is very high or low in the sky. Taking note of these details creates greater interest in the ball. You may discover darker places on your courts, where the lights don't have full effect, improving your night time play with better awareness of the challenges you face at a particular court.

## Riding with the Ball

This one might seem a little strange for some people, but imagine you are riding on the ball. Imagine the perspective of what you would experience, if you were sitting on top of it, as it flew to the other side of the court. Helping people learn to shift perspective away from their exact location can help them in many instances.

**Players can start to see more tactical advantages, when they shift their awareness to, what is happening on the other side of the court.**

Doing this, also helps you discover, what are your opponent's least favorite shots. Certain speeds, heights, arcs, spins might cause them to make errors, or hit less aggressively, and you then have something you can use in a tight spot. In the short term, this may take away focus from performing a proper follow through, finishing to your stroke, but then you may want to shift to having this experience, in your imagination, and that can enhance your ability to hit targets on the court as well.

### Paying Attention only to the Arc of the Shot

Every ball has a different arc in which it travels. Take time to be fascinated by those trajectories. One of the coolest things about ball sports, is that the ball never comes the same way twice. Part of what makes tennis the best sport in the world, is that the player gets to interact with the ball many more times in competition, than any other sport, thus increasing the influence of visual decision making, on the outcome of the match. Before playing only two set matches became common place, the average number of hits, by a player, in a match was 487. I use this as a motivational tool for my players to fall in love with the sport.

### Where else are you going to hit the ball 487 times?

As stated previously, bringing our mind's attention to different and more specific details of the ball and its flight, assists in either the ability to focus, or to use our peripheral vision. For example, if we ask a player to find the logo on the ball in flight, that is a focus drill, because it falls within the 3 degree window of focus. This activity is a peripheral vision/tracking exercise. Seeing the arc of the ball, and noticing how the arc of every ball is different every shot, challenges us to use peripheral vision to track the ball, and this is done with a relatively still head.

Forty-Five

# On Court Visual Challenge Drills (Part Four)
# Tactical Awareness in Space

*Beginners and low intermediates will struggle to perform these drills. Anyone who wants to be advanced or an elite competitor must become excellent at them. From these basic drills it's not hard to come up with many variations that can work for you.*
*~ BP*

### Predicting: Height Over Net

A fun activity to perform with fairly high skilled players, among tournament junior players, and adults 3.5 and above, is to have them predict how high over the net the ball will cross, and do so as close to the time, of the opponent's ball strike is possible.

**This is very challenging observation and decision making drill, and very difficult to do with 100% accuracy.**

You might not want to do this for more than 5 minutes, calling out the number of feet over the net, but then once the exercise has been done, the player's minds should be interested in looking for that for a period of time after then exercise is over. I don't recommend immediately shifting to a new exercise, give players up to 10 minutes to internalize the experience.

### Predicting: Zone on Court, or Zone of Hit

As a coach, you define your zones on court according to your own program, so I will leave it up to you to design this, but it will be challenging for players to predict the zone where the ball will bounce prior to the opponent's ball crossing the net. Also, different coaches define zones of receiving the ball with different systems, ABCD, 123, 1234, with different reference points of below the knee, above or below the hips, or shoulders, etc.

**Add a prediction of ball reception height, prior to the ball crossing the net.**

The next step up would be for a player to call out where they want to hit their shot before the ball crosses the net using options like Loop, Drive, Drop, Slice, or Dip, or whatever terminology you use for different spin and placement options. Depending on style of play, you may also want to include a rule that a player will not address the same type of shot twice. You can use this to build better disguise of your shots, into your game.

### Predicting Zone of Position in Court to Receive

Another subtle ball recognition exercise is for players to predict where on the court they will be standing when they receive the ball. One of the cool things that happens between the last three exercises explained is the variability from ball to ball. Almost never will a player take the ball in the same reception zone, standing in the same zone, with the ball landing in the same zone two times in a row. Making predictions on other parts of the performance may have to wait, but try to predict well before the ball crosses the net.

**This may be hard for some players, but the prediction skills may cause a challenge in brain activity to develop the capacity.**

Younger and more inexperienced players might have a delay in the verbal processing, which does not allow them to make the prediction before the ball crosses the net, so use your best judgement. Getting impatient with yourself or others on this task, will not help anything. Taking video from the net post, can help determine how well and early players are performing the task. It's best if the coach can give immediate correction to errors in judgement. Using video from behind the student can also help them see in slow motion what actually happened, raising their ability to recognize the ball in new ways.

### Variations

You can use marked balls, colored targets, marked off zones in the court, or any number of visual cues or targets to create a decision making game or exercise. I like to make ideal zones worth more points, certain balls marked a certain way must be struck to a certain place, get creative.

Note: keep in mind that its good to use only one word, or come up with another way to express the decision for those who are slow verbal processors. I recommend NOT criticizing yourself or others if you are not as fast at producing the word that expresses the decision, as long as you can make the visual decision immediately as it becomes available.

Forty-Six

## Use Objective Observations Of Your Shot Placements

*'You have described only too well,' replied the Master, 'where the difficulty lies... The right shot at the right moment does not come because you do not let go of yourself. You...brace yourself for failure. So long as that is so, you have no choice but to call forth something yourself that ought to happen independently of you, and so long as you call it forth your hand will not open in the right way--like the hand of a child.'*
~ *(Zen and the Art of Archery)*

Players make great gains, when they discover the true landing place of their shots. This differs from what they formerly perceived, as the location of their shot, in the court. As a player is beginning to make the transition, from subjective to more accurate objective evaluation of shots, they move from intermediate to advanced player. The ability to hit balls to smaller target areas of the court, becomes much more important, as you go up the levels. As the refinement of this mental faculty improves, practicing and improving shot accuracy can also improve.

**The problem for many players, is that they believe they are hitting a target area in competition, when in reality, they are not.**

This also happens in drill situations, even when the stress level of the drill is much lower than actual competition. Part of the solution, is to create challenges for the eyes and brain to properly measure and approach higher levels of precision. Having clearly marked target areas, that are a realistic size, to allow for some success supports confidence. Using a dead center bullseye target, to get your mind interested in the center of that area is a best practice in task creation.

So, when missing the bullseye still equates to making a shot in the larger acceptable target you have the concept of 'hitting to big targets'. Even so, it's proper use of the eyes, and the mind/body connection, that will make for better performance. When introduced to the challenge of really seeing how their target hitting performance actually is, most players are confronted with the fact that they have a lot of room for improvement, in this aspect of their game.

**Almost universally, players feel some internal pressure to perform, even when there is no external pressure to do so, simply a zone or area to hit into on the other side confronting them.**

People have to be presented with a something to aim at, for them to understand how, having a target has them feeling inside. How you approach that leads to an exploration of the mind/body connection. Players tend initially to try too hard to aim, hitting targets, then tense up, and become frustrated. Now let's move more into the process, of perfecting ability to hit the ball where you want.

## Mind/Body Performance

Teaching the mind/body connection, when it comes to hitting a target is a part of the fundamental training of any player. It's best to introduce objects, for which to aim shots, early in the process of learning the game. The human brain is still the most powerful computer processor in the world, and amazing processing can happen when we learn to get out of the way of what our brain, eyes and hand can do, when learning naturally, how to place a ball. Allowing for discovery, about how your eyes and brain cooperate, to make adjustments to your performance, can set you on a path to much higher levels of play.

### Good Shot > Bad Shot > Tension > Frustration > Repeat

First, we move away from subjectively judging our shots as 'good' or 'bad'. When we hit a 'good' shot, then we immediately feel pressure to do it again. A large group of my students in their first lessons are stuck on knowing 'How did I do that?'. And then when thinking those thoughts indirectly leads to missing the next one, or are least not performing the shot with the same smoothness and accuracy, they develop their mental emotional complex over, their perceived inability to hit two good shots in a row.

**Do you, like many others, have an internal dialogue after hitting one nice shot, then one not so nice one, asking themselves 'Why can't I do it twice in a row?'**

When we hit a 'bad' shot, our social training and self talk generally says to 'analyze what went wrong and try harder'. We have to step out of this negative cycle. It's in the trying harder, that we find an increase in tension, which then blocks better performances. I often see a good shot, followed by a bad shot, followed by a worse shot created by too much tension, which leads to frustration, and maybe an accidental good shot, then the process repeats, and might deepen.

## Learning To Make Objective Observations

The better you are at objectively observing what you are doing, and it's effect on the ball, the better able you will be able to learn on the day how to hit ht shots you want. Moving toward a modality of seeing and feeling what is happening, rather than trying to think your way through is most helpful, but it might not yet be a well developed modality of 'thought' for you. It's not traditional Western thinking. Setting aside thoughts that take you away from actually seeing and feeling the results of our shots, taking note of exactly how far the shot is from the target, opens up in our mind, a window to allow our brain and body, to collaborate better to produce better results.

**The reality of vision, is that most of the impulses, that create our visual experience, come from inside the brain.**

As we have discussed, a small percentage of your vision, comes through your eyes right now. Most of it is in your brain and imagination from your stored memories. So, we must mindfully leave that mode in practice, arriving at an actual time of observing how far the ball was from the target. Once we do that, then our brain gets busy, making minute adjustments, to move the next shot closer to the target.

## Good Shot = Pressure < 4.5

A common cycle I see with players below a 4.5 level is acknowledgement of a good shot, or even great shot, which then leads to a feeling of pressure 'Can I do it again' seems to be the internal message. Another outcome is the elation which comes from a dose of Dopamine in the brain, causing the feelings of euphoria. My experience tells me that moments after the elation, vision is clouded and people become momentarily uncoordinated from the Dopamine fix.

**The elation over the 'good' shot, compromises the ability to hit the next shot, which is often 'bad'.**

As this cycle plays out over a period of time, it's easy for us to develop a belief system about how permanent this problem might be. I get players who say, 'I have a bad backhand.' The meaning of which is that they own their backhand, and it's a permanent problem that they need solved. I start them off with the idea that they used to have a bad backhand, and now they are learning a better one.

Addressing the deep seated belief, that they can't hit two great shots in a row, or that they always miss on the third one, is not easy, but it is simple. What they really need, is to learn to accept that they can hit two good shots in a row, if they delay gratification after the first one, taking a deep breath between points resetting themselves for the beginning of the next point. How many times have you seen an ace, followed up by a double fault in lower level play? These internal dialogues take up energy, and they exist in a modality of thought that takes a subjectively judgmental approach, which makes using the proper modality for seeing and hitting a target more difficult.

## How To Get Fully Objective

What is the answer? Learn to put away subjective judgements about shots. Don't call them good or bad, and if you are expressing emotions over shots, then listen to whether those are connected to subjective judgements. It's hard to say that you aren't thinking it was a bad shot, if you are growling. Eliminate any subjective description of a shot. Instead, use your eyes to simply measure:

'10 feet to the right, and 5 feet too far.'
'10 feet to the left, and 3 feet too far.'
'5 feet to the right, and 2 feet short'
'3 feet left and 1 foot short'
'1 foot right, and 1 foot far'

You will start to see a refinement, and then as soon as you get too excited by the process of improvement, then it will all fall apart and you have to go back to the process of simple, emotionless, looking at the result of the shot.

Where there are overcompensations, they are compensations nonetheless. Accept those, because it's the natural learning taking place. When this happens with my players, I ask them to hit something in the middle of the two previous shots. Over 90% of the time they can, which shows learning. Sometimes their shot is very close to the middle of the last two shots, but sometimes only marginally so, but any progress is good progress. Approximately 20% of the time, the player will hit a ball almost precisely between the last two missed shots. In essence, players need to get out of the way, of their own brain.

## Stay In The Process

Stay with the process of marking the location of each shot, by placing another ball in the place that it landed, until 20 or 30 shots have been made. Try to identify a pattern. Ask the player what triggers them. Many times a ball very close to the target gets very exciting, and then you have that Dopamine again. I believe you can clear it out with one breath, but I have no hard science on that. Depending on how the player is responding it may be good to clear the 20 or 30 balls to start fresh, and observe if the next grouping looks better. As in archery, or shooting, we look for groupings of shots, rather than absolute accuracy at first. It's nice to say, 'OK, you seem to have a grouping that is a little short and to the left, so now hit a little further and to the right.'

Forty-Seven

## What Are The Next Steps In Hitting More Targets Better?

*Every Shot Must Be Hit With A Target In Mind.*
*~ A Tennis Maxim*

### Trust Your Brain

The largest percentage of the brain's activity lies in your vision, which is among the unspoken unseen workings of controlling the unconscious processes, that keep your body alive. The great power of this unconscious play, is on full display when we watch the best players in the world. A recent study showed anecdotally, the difference between the brain activity of a novice at work compared to a master. The masterful performer had far less brain activity when performing the task than the novice. Additionally, there was evidence to suggest that certain activities had become hardwired in the synaptical connections of the performer.

**In essence, the performance becomes part of the person.**

The master owns the movement. When players are very ambitious and willful, they often times try so hard that they introduce tension in their muscles, and subjective judgements in their mind, which takes up conflicting and not very helpful brain power, they are simply working against what can happen very naturally, and with much more ease. So, instead of owning a flowing shot that shows maximum efficiency, they buy one that gives them tension, frustration, and just frequently enough good shots to keep them seeking The Holy Grail - consistency.

### Martial Arts Parable

The student came to the master asking, 'Master, how long until I can be a master like you?'. The Master replied, '10 years'. The student proclaimed their diligence and that they would work twice as hard as others, putting twice the amount of time into the task. The Master hearing this said. '20 years'.

So, instead of focusing so much on working hard, players can shift to quieting the mind, leaving the complications of hard work, coming completely to seeing exactly what is. As players develop a more accurate understanding, of how a certain shot feels, when it goes to the target area, and continue to play, until more and more consecutive repetitions allow for the ball to be hit in the target area, then that can be even further developed, into even greater accuracy. Too much 'work' clouds the mind, the vision, and gets in the way of the natural learning process.

## Hitting Where You Want

Many times when watching professional players in practice, I have marveled at how some great players use 30 to 60 minutes hitting ONE type of shot and doing so with remarkable accuracy. Any blip of the radar of missing the target is wiped out of the mind and the process begins again of finding the target and hitting it repeatedly. That level of precision is only really possible with impeccable vision, and the relaxation of purpose, to do it repeatedly.

Over the years I have read articles from journalists who have taken the time to hit with professional players at the very top of the game. Perhaps the professionals took it easy on the journalist (the ones I know are around 4.5 level), but the common thread, in the reporting of the experience has been, that they were much more impressed with player's ability to hit the ball anywhere they want on the court, more so than the power of their shots.

No matter what style of play you use, accuracy of shot is vital to success, if you can't hit it where you want with enough regularity, you will be on the losing end. To do that end, the visual training is much more connected to the mind/body experience of learning to hit a target.

Forty-Eight

# Why Will The Visual And Kinesthetic Always Be Intertwined?

*Instead of reality being passively recorded
by the brain, it is actively constructed by it.*
~ David Eagleman

A second anecdote, from the aforementioned BBC special, on The Brain sheds light on the experience of visual learning. David Eagleman participated in a study where his vision was purposely distorted. The test used special mirrors and lenses, to completely turn his visual experience from right to left, to left to right. The show's host, then had to learn to do everything opposite, of what his previous training had been. In his discussion with the researcher heading the project, he was advised that he should touch everything in his surroundings. He then he would have better mental markers as a frame of reference for his visual decision making. How will we make this practical in the sports world? We can go about constructing a reality that fits as accurately as possible with what is really happening.

Like the sniper, who imagines that he has a hand in his mind, that drops the bullet two miles away at the target, you might have your own unique mental construction, for how this process works for you. The use of the word hand is interesting, because it meshes with the true nature of tennis. Raq in Eqyptian means palm, and that is the root of Racquet, and tennis originated from Jeu de Palm which was a royal game of hand ball. When you imagine your strings, as a hand for catching and tossing, you can better use the implement to throw the ball where you want.

## Outside In - The Visual Field

In the experience of playing tennis, but also other sports, the experience of feeling the shot, knowing proprioceptive position in space, is required to advance in the sport. Knowledge of where you are in the court, and what that does to your options for shot making, can make all the difference in your tactical play. Pairing vision and the kinesthetic experience is vital for the full understanding of the visual, knowing where you are, and connecting that to what you feel in your frame.

**The confusion that comes from a shift in vision, or a lack of familiarity with our surroundings makes brain work much harder to see.**

We become much more reliant on our eyes, when our surroundings are less familiar, because our brain has less on record, in our mind, of what exists in that space. This is one reason why it's easier to play in familiar surroundings, and less so in strange or different ones. It's a good idea to arrive early at a new site to take in the sights and sounds of the new place.

### Inside Out - The Contact Point

For this reason, I work very hard, with newer players, to establish their understanding of the contact point. Seeing, feeling, knowing their contact point, the most important place and time in tennis, is critical to their future success in the sport. I see so many players who have modern technique, but have substandard awareness of the contact point, and many times they lose to those whose strokes are not as developed, but do have their contact point dialed in to their game. The issue that affects tennis players the most, is a lack of awareness of what they are doing. They don't tune into how it feels, to do what they are doing on a tennis court.

**These issues are many times resolved by, pairing the video of what that the player is doing, with the guided experience of how they approach or swing.**

They can also begin to see how they swing to and through the ball , compared with the ideal stroke that we want to teach. In one of my favorite interviews, that I have conducted on my former podcast, I asked Torben Ulrich about how someone best learns to play tennis, his answer in his Danish accent, 'Well Bill, I think you need to know what you are doing'. This one piece of advice can take quite a while to unpack, and seems to be among the best pieces of advice anyone could ever gain. 'How can you make a change in what you are doing, if you don't know what are you doing? How will you know if the change is in effect, and is relatively permanent if you don't know what you are doing?' The knowing of what we are doing is predicated on a more accurate ability to objectively observe it.

### Variability of Conditions: Making Adjustments

One tricky item that is most understood by players at 4.5 and above, is that players often do not feel the same from day to day, match to match. They may be hot or cold, they could be experiencing stiffness in one area of their body, their energy level may be high or low, all of this can have an effect on how they experience their shots.

The difference in the conditions, such as how much do the balls bounce, the speed of the court, the position of the sun in the sky, how hot or how cold it is, and finally the wind have an effect on the visual and kinesthetic experience of the player.

Great players know that they have to learn, how to play in the conditions of the day. These factors have an impact on your visual experience of the ball. People many times assume that play tennis is a uniform experience, and that everything should be the same, but all the above factors make a difference in how your playing will meet the new visual challenge.

## Understand The Subtleties Of Conditions

The Inuit people are said to have 5,000 words for snow. I'm not sure if thats true, but you might imagine they many ways to describe it by necessity. Tennis players and coaches might also need a deep lexicon to describe conditions that will effect the visual experience. Quite commonly lower level players have pretty strong negative reactions to conditions that are out of their comfort zone, commonly that means hating the wind. As players improve and gain a wealth of experience, we as coaches can help them solve one problem at a time such as: 'Here is what to do when the sun is in your eyes,' Or 'When the wind is like this, you can expect that.' When my players have had a negative experience in the wind, then we have a wind lesson. I generally don't teach when conditions are so blustery that the ball is going everywhere, but when I have a player who really needs to learn how to deal with it, then we do the lesson.

**One of the truly exciting things about tennis is the myriad of problems that players experience, and that may explain why psychological studies of tennis players, point to them being the best problem solvers in sports.**

So, ultimately, using a pairing of visual ability and tactile awareness, every problem may be solved one at a time. I know some courts where the surface was not applied very well, a little uneven in terms of the sand in the mixture of the paint, and then over time as the courts wore down, there were some very smooth parts, and some very rough parts of the court surface. This made the ball fairly unpredictable, as when it hit a smooth part, the ball stayed faster and low. When a ball hit a rough part or a crack, it would slow down and maybe jump up seemingly. Seeing the bounce of the ball was a huge key in playing on that surface. Every surface is unique, because no two court resurfacing jobs are exactly the same. Nicer clubs tend to have the most uniform playing surface, but you can find small areas where the ball plays differently, a slight undulation in the court and the ball can jump in a different direction by a few inches, enough to make your contact point less than ideal. Whenever you go a new court, be sure to inspect it for cracks, bumps, undulations, etc. You then can be better prepared for the visual challenges of the day.

Forty-Nine

# Why You Should Bring Your Ruler To The Court To Measure The Ball

*Use the tennis racquet to measure your shots.*
*~ Unknown*

'Get your Racquet Back' might be among the worst things a coach can say, and this mostly for visual training reasons. It lacks specificity of time and location. When do you do it? How far back? When my racquet is back, I can no longer see it. The best players in the world, actually delay their backswing, until the last possible moment, this helps them to create maximum racquet head speed, manage the size of their backswing.

## How To Measure Your Movement

Instead, use your racquet as a measuring stick. The pairing of the tip of the racquet, with the track of the incoming ball, is among the most important skills, for gaining proper position with the ball. The contact point is always the most important moment in tennis, but setting your racquet to the side, to allow you to measure your footwork, is vital to learning great positioning for the ball. Players who remain facing forward too long, then turn and get the racquet back all at once, find themselves often too close, and alternately too far away from the ball.

**Generally, each player has a tendency to either be too close or too far away, so it makes sense to figure out which one is your tendency, and solve that problem first, then move on to solving the other one.**

There was a young lady who was getting ready to play at the University of Texas, who when she hit the ball at one particular location, hit amazingly powerful and accurate shots, but when she took the ball just a few inches further away, then she lost some power and control. It was in dialing in the contact, with just a bit more accuracy, which created an amazing jump, in her efficiency of shot. Taking one more small step to get laser accuracy to her footwork, allowed her to raise her game another full step.

## Ready, Measure, Slot, Contact

What is the Measuring Position? The racquet tip is up, in front of the player, angled slightly forward, although some top players might even angle their racquet 30 degrees forward in the preparation phase of the stroke. Go look at some video! With a turn of the body approximately 45 degrees to the side, you are now prepared for a screamer to come at you and using all of it's pace to bunt it back, or you can read the call coming more slowly rotating up to another 45 degrees or more to generate the power you need. ( Many players rely too much on their arm to develop power).

**Players who have their racquet back too early cannot pair their racquet with the ball as easily, and are prone to fail at getting into ideal position to strike the ball, on balance with a clean shot, with good posture.**

Often those same players will make last minute lunges to the ball, or find them selves too close, needing to back away from the ball, throwing them off balance. As players advance they may tilt the frame slightly forward to help facilitate racquet head speed. One thought that sometimes helps players is the idea of throwing the tip of the racquet at the ball, but be careful as it won't work with everyone, so it might not be for you, but it has helped me and others.

## 1,2,3 Contact Targets

With intermediates and below, adequate ball spacing can be difficult. Having players self evaluate after their shots really helps. So we call it a '1,' if the player is too close to the ball, and a '3' if they are too far, but a '2' when they are in a comfortable zone and can take an easy swing. After a few minutes, or even a few sessions of this exercise, we might start to say 2.5, 1.8, 2.2, and refine their understanding of ideal spacing. For a 2, they must be on balance, with good posture, ball in the center of the strings, without abnormal reaching to the ball with the arm. Over time, players discover that, if they use more precise movements, then they get the ball in their strings more efficiently. This is something they must experience visually and using the racquet to measure the space, brings more awareness to ideal distance to contact point.

Fifty

## Using Slow Motion Video to Support Visual Awareness

*Slow motion goes one of two ways. It either makes it look really, really cool, or it makes it look really, really bad.*
*~ Blake Griffin*

This week on an internet coach's forum, there was an interesting conflict, in regard to the use of slow motion video. A few very smart coaches banded together to say that their eyes are so good, that they don't need video to show them what is really happening. As an occasional contractor of super slow motion video services in 2011 with a friend who owned a cutting edge camera, we would video the players at my club in super slow motion. We were crestfallen when just 18 months later this technology became widely available, and we could no longer host special stroke clinics that were unique in the industry. Even though the enticement to see themselves play in slow motion is gone, people are still not using the amazing cameras on their phones and tablets enough. Phones seem to be ahead of tablets at this time offering even 4k. You don't need 4k, but what you really want is frames per second.

**Some cameras will easily do 120 FPS, some will do 240 FPS which is a bit of overkill, but you can get a bit more detail, even though playback will be half as fast.**

You can also find camera apps, for your phone, that record in 60 fps, which give you the ability to advance the playback on a slide bar, going frame by frame forward and backward. The truth is that the coaches above could not possibly have seen well enough, even with their trained eyes, to capture what a slow motion camera can show. My eyes were opened to a hidden world, and my foggy perceptions of what was happening, were cleared up, allowing me understand where breakdowns occur, and help players understand the subtleties of refined technique.

Vic Braden said that the best angle to film a student is from behind, because you capture the player's same visual field of reference, and the player then can see the mysterious actions of their body, arm and racquet that happen behind them in the same direction as their point of view. This works very well to pair the visual with the kinesthetic experience of the shot.

## Various Filming Angles

I also like to film from 45 degrees in front of a player, to see how well they make contact on the 45 degree plane, away from them. Jack Broudy has been a pioneer in addressing the more or less ideal contact point approximately 45 degrees in front of us. Contact me to get in touch with Jack's new tennis teaching system that will be launching in 2021.

**I also do some video taping from the side at 90 degrees, as this perspective allows us to see more of the different phases of the swing.**

The other two angles show me much more of what I want my players to understand. Far too often tennis coaches use only video taken from 90 degrees. On serves ,it can be helpful also to take vide from behind the student at 90 degrees along the baseline as well, because there is a lot that happens with the hand and frame behind the player.

Keep in mind that some players will not allow you to film them at all, and you must ask permission of a parent before filming a child.

## Three Angles Of Viewing Or More

When a stroke is particularly troublesome, it can be a good idea to look at it from as many angles as possible. A great example of this is some video of one of my favorite fast rising players on the ATP tour, from 2018, who happens to have a fantastic backhand, but a forehand that was less than 100% accurate. Since I wrote this about Alexander Zverev, he has a much improved forehand and is now a solid top ten player, who looks like a Grand Slam winner sometime in the next few years. A year ago, I had seen his stroke from various angles, but when I saw a particular video shot from 45 degrees away from his backhand side, which showed his backhand and a few forehands, a peculiar and variable preparation of the racquet, on the forehand side became quite obvious to me.

**The point being that sometimes taking time on a troublesome stroke to look from various vantage points can really help in understanding a stroke, that cannot be done from the normal perspectives of playing or coaching.**

The more you can create something approaching 3 dimensional constructs, the more likely you are to see the root of a perplexing problem. It runs counter culture, to look at things from different perspectives. The visual challenges of coaching can be as difficult as playing. As a player a best practice is to hire a coach who looks at your game closely, or take the video yourself from at least 2 angles to see what you can.

## SwingVision Is A Game Changer

SwingVision will also come in handy, because you can split out only the real play, finding the precise shots that give you trouble, you can look at the shots you made with a certain shot, and the shots you missed. What I recommend is that you sign up for the free version, play around with it, then when you are ready to get full use of the Pro version come back to the link and do it when you are sure you can maximize it's use. Yes, if you subscribe then I get some compensation. So, if you support getting the visual tennis message out there, then subscribing will definitely help.

Fifty-One

# Is Anticipation Really Possible? How To Read And React Without The Guesswork

*A great source of calamity lies in regret and anticipation; therefore a person is wise who thinks of the present alone, regardless of the past or future.*
~ Oliver Goldsmith

It's important to understand anticipation on a tennis court, what it is, and what it is not. I prefer not to use that word, instead the phrase 'Understanding The Opponent's Tendencies' is far better, because there can still be a few options. Some people interpret anticipation to mean, guessing what they opponent will hit ahead of time. That leads to moving for the wrong shot, when you infer incorrectly. Having the presence of mind, and clarity, to objectively observe your opponent's likely shot or shots in certain situations prepares you better to read and react. This is where a measured amount of thinking, and the taking of mental notes between points, with a little self talk thrown in, can educate your eyes, aiding in decision making.

## Read and React: Take Mental Notes

What we have learned about how vision is processed in the brain, would seem to confirm that a mindful approach to understanding the opponent is paramount. Taking mental notes, by saying things to yourself like, 'when I hit my approach shot low to his backhand he seems to try to thread the needle down the line,' or 'she hits her first passing shot, almost always crosscourt'. If you try to anticipate ahead of the play, without taking notice of the other player's habits, you can be susceptible to the opponent's 'change up' play.

It's a great idea to play certain patterns long enough for the opponent to start to think they can anticipate your shots. Then, after setting them up with one shot, use a different smart shot, that is one you haven't you haven't shown them before. This keeps them guessing and thus delays their reaction time with more thought, but only if you have developed a pattern for them to follow. However, you don't want to fall into the same trap that you set for others. Advanced players, when they get a short ball, out of 10 shots, they can approach the net to the backhand 7 times (crosscourt or down the line), to the forehand one time, attempt a drop shot one time, and go for a short angle winner one time.

**If you only came to the net, 10 times out of 10, on those opportunities, and did not mix it up, then you might run the risk of giving your opponent practice in beating you.**

This is true if they are wanting to come to the net often. The advantage gained by switching up the play, is that the opponent has to use part of their reaction time, seeing the ball, deciding what you are doing, then reacting. They will not be able to immediately react to a net approach. One of the most effective ways to stretch the court, and throw a wrench into your opponent's anticipation, is when instead of hitting an approach to the backhand, you hit a drop shot to the forehand, thus creating the furthest run, from the area they anticipated you might be hitting your approach shot. You accomplish two things: 1. You slow down the other player's reactions, and 2. You give them a much wider area of the court to defend.

### Take The Notes, But Learn To Wait

Turn this around in your mind, be the opponent, learn to wait, read and react and do so quickly. This is why it's very important to see the ball and your opponent's racquet interacting on the other side of the court, to give your eyes all the necessary information to make a proper read. Training your ability to wait, to pay attention to your opponent's shot, on a moment to moment basis, is a key indicator to success. Additionally, you will get better at knowing your opponent's options for shot making on any particular shot you hit, and you can start to see how they tip you off before lobs, drop shots, and other tricky shots.

**It is wise to be on the lookout, to react quickly to the shot, that will put you under pressure.**

For instance, if you come to the net, be quick to read a lob, so you can be ready to immediately hit an overhead. If you are first aware of the lob, then you can develop a lot of confidence coming forward, because being lobbed successfully is one of the fears of the net rusher. Your ability to read and react to a lob will decrease the percentage of successful lobs against you. Of course, nothing will protect you from a perfect lob to the baseline. Learn to prioritize the read of the shot that can hurt you the worst.

To conclude, read, react and train your instincts!

Fifty-Two

# How To Prepare Your Eyes For Competition Without Sapping Your Energy

*Failure to prepare, is preparing to fail.*
*~ General George S. Patton*

When preparing to play, there are a few things you can do to give your eyes an advantage. Develop a routine from about 45 minutes before your match time where you let yourself quiet down, and get very calm mentally and emotionally. A physical warm up, along with some static and dynamic stretching can get you ready for fast action on court, but can also reduce your physical tension and stress. Stretching time is also a great time to bring your brain speed down for more clarity.

**Take it slow when warming up on court, make your first priority picking up the ball on time.**

Have a ball awareness drill, that is your go to, that you will perform for the first few minutes of your warm up, then internalize it. Even before your warm up time, if you haven't been to the tournament site before, walk around and get familiar with the place, and look for possible distractions, like low walls that ricochet balls onto other courts and the like. If you can scout a possible future opponent, that can be good, or find the best played match you can find and take a look at that for a few minutes. Do a fast reaction drill with BlazePods, Q-Ball, Z-Ball or another reaction time aid.

## Action Items for Your Eyes

1. **Warm them up properly**. Start with some easy shots and give yourself a few minutes to shift from scanning and tracking to focusing on the ball.

2. **Fine tune your focus** using any number of ball awareness drills, choose your favorite.

3. **Watch your opponent**. Notice the subtle differences in their stroke, or timing that leads to a cross court ball, down the line, higher or lower ball, or different spins. Try to find their idiosyncrasy or something that gives away

where they are hitting.

4. If you can't watch your opponent in a match, it's very important to observe them closely in the **5 minute warm up**. Find out if they look at the place they will hit before they do, many players telegraph their shots with their eyes ahead of time, especially on serve.

5. You can **use a reaction ball** like a Q-ball, or a Z-ball to warm up your eyes. A regular ball will seem easy after that. Hitting volleys with the tiny keychain stress ball also gets you seeing quite well, and you can do that in a parking lot, if there are no courts available for warm up.

Fifty-Three

# Is Being 'Always On' A Good Idea?
# How To Diminish Mental Visual Fatigue

*Fatigue makes cowards of us all.*
*~ Winston Churchill*

Everyone has a limited ability to concentrate for long periods of time. The average attention span is 15 minutes, but even though tennis players are much above that, I can promise you it's very likely you will have some minor dip in concentration about every 45 minutes. Beginner players may be able to focus for a few points, then lose focus, regain it, lose it and so on... Advancing players will be able to concentrate for longer periods of time, until they have a break in their attention span.

**World Class players may be able to concentrate up to and beyond 6 hours with limited breaks in concentration.**

When those disruptions in their full attention occur, they are potentially the deciding factor in a match. In reality, world ranked players are able to concentrate for much longer periods of time overall, largely because they don't try to concentrate at every moment. And the behavior they exhibit with their eyes is a large part of that.

## Professionals Avoid 'Always On' Behavior

Watch carefully any professional player, and the attention to a ball during the point, each player will have full concentration just prior to the toss going up in the air. Sometimes you will see a player open their eyes very wide prior to the beginning of a point. Djokovic does this in a big way, quite often ahead of big points. The point is played, then almost immediately each player will allow their eyes to rest. Watch some points in slow motion, looking for the shift between ON and OFF. They let their body go relaxed, eyes go into soft focus, they will take a relaxed walk to prepare for the next point.

Close your eyes for a moment, then ask your self to rest your eyes. If you are holding onto any tension behind your eyes let it go. Soft eyes, is a great phrase, you can use, during breaks in the action to remind yourself to let go of tension. Most likely, the act of closing your eyes helped, but the act of giving your eyes permission to rest can like a deeper level of relaxation.

## 16 Second Cure

In Jim Loehr's '16 second cure,' one of the seminal pieces of practical Sport Psychology, he gives advice for players to maximize the largest time segment of the match, the time between points. It's how you manage this time that will tell quite a bit about how you are managing your anxiety, intensity, relaxation, and recovery.

## The Decisive Stage

The first objective is to acknowledge that the previous point is over, this allows you to move past it, because you created closure. This is called The Decisive Stage, meaning that the point has been decided, so that outcome will not change. You immediately acknowledge and accept the end of that point. At that moment, one-second avert your gaze, look in a dramatically different direction, as the physical act of turning, helps foster the mental emotional act of leaving that point behind.

**Your eyes can help create a strong body language effect, saying non-verbally, that the point is behind you.**

Of course, if there is some reason to linger, than do so, like, if your opponent made a bad call. You might want to take a nice long stare at the line. If your opponent is asking you a question, of course you give them eye contact. After that, it's time to transition forward, into the other steps of the cure.

## Relaxation Stage

Next up, is the relaxation stage, which includes maybe a deep breath, maybe scanning through your body for tension and releasing it. Most importantly, resting your eyes on an object, your racquet strings, the court, something, or just closing them for one-second. If you feel nervous, it's a great idea to make sure you take at least one deep breath between points, your nervous system needs oxygen, and you can calm your nerves with good breathing. If you feel like you can't take a deep breath, then try emptying all the air out of your lungs as much as you can first, this will make more room for the air coming into your lungs.

**Passively, let go of any residual tension in your eyes, go 'soft focus', until such time as you are in the Ritual Phase.**

Practice resting your eyes between points, and you most likely find that you can concentrate during points for a longer period of time. I strongly recommend that your eyes rest on only a few things between points: the ball, your frame, the ground or your opponent. It can be a good idea to check in on your competitor's body language to look for signs of weakness, or to find out what kind of battle you are facing. Unless there is a very good reason, do not look outside the four fences of the court, as it's highly likely that you will become visually distracted by something or someone outside your court.

## The Preparation Stage

The third stage of Loehr's cure is The Preparation Stage where you are advised, to quickly take stock of what happened, in the previous point and definitely plan the next point according to your game plan. This is also a great time to develop empowering self talk, saying a certain word or two. I recommend 'I can do this', but you might have a phrase from this book as to good words to use as visual cues like 'read and react,' 'only the ball' or a phrase of your making. As we have discovered in the different facets of this book, everything Loehr suggests will be helpful in processing the visual input that was gained in the previous point.

**This is where the work you have done to develop your imagination, through visualization will pay off.**

One thing I know from 30 years of coaching, is that some people have a better capacity to create a visual image in their mind of what has just happened, few seem to be almost devoid of that ability, but it is something that can be practiced and improved. Close your eyes, and remember the best point you can remember, that you have played in your life so far, you can likely conjure up how it ended. For me, it was on center court at a club, and on match point at full extension, I made a deft drop volley winner, at full stretch, with a crowd watching, and a few people even clapped for me. So few of our matches finish, with a great shot, people watching and appreciating it.

Allowing yourself to let down and relax in the Relaxation Phase, also facilitates being able to go into your mind and imagination, for a moment. There is danger here, DO NOT start analyzing your strokes too much, but simply make a note of what just happened, and how do you want to respond. Maybe you did hit in the net, and you need to take a practice stroke for how you would lift that ball up the next time, the pairing of the visual and kinesthetic in a practice shot can be the programming you need to break up a bad pattern.

**Your sole objective in going to your mind is to draw on the memory of what happened, so that you can objectively observe it and adjust your play accordingly.**

This allows you to take a more rational view of what is really going on in the match. If you are carrying mounting stress, then it can be more difficult to see what is going on, as your judgement may be clouded with anxiety. Of all the stages The Relaxation Stage might be most important for this reason. But the final one, might be the second most important.

## The Ritual Stage

Finally, the last stage of the 16 second cure is called The Ritual Stage, where you have a routine action or short set of actions, that you always do the same way. Loehr recommends going into your automatic ritual for serve and return. Having a visual aspect to your ritual can be important also, having certain places you look, or don't look, as you prepare for a point. For your serve, a great thing to do is to look at your target, but also look at a place in the service box that is NOT your target.

**I have noticed opponents that tip off their serve location, during their pre-serve ritual, by only looking at the place they want to serve to, making it much easier to return.**

As you improve, you can simply visualize your target in your mind, without directly looking at the court, this helps you avoid giving away your intentions to your opponent. On return, you want to remind yourself to see the ball from the opponent's contact point, and it's not helpful to follow the toss upward. The change of direction from the toss going up, to the contact point of the serve, makes it more tricky to follow. For the purposes of using your eyes just enough and not tiring them out, you can get your eyes to the anticipated contact point at the moment that the toss is initiated. Once the point has begun, then you will go into the flow, of the system of your visual skills, subconsciously transitioning from one skill to another as previously discussed. If you notice a break down, then you might want to make your preparation phrase to 'see the ball out of their strings', or 'focus from the bounce', or something else that works for you.

## A Bad Break In Ritual

On a humorous note, in practice situations, I find that when one of my players looks at me, while they are in the middle of their service motion, that they have about a 5% serve percentage on those attempts. I teach them not to allow themselves, to be distracted by looking at anything, but the ball during their service motion.

## It's OK To Close Your Eyes

You need to know what works for you between points to rest your eyes, including even closing them for a moment, but when you are entering back into a concentrated mode into the point, make sure your eyes are set for maximum concentration with zero distractions.

Fifty-Four

## Is It Really Possible To Be Perfectly Level Headed?  How To Use Ideal Posture For Visual Acuity

*When things are steep,
remember to stay level headed.*
~ Horace

One of the most common issues players have, is that they put their body into strange, off balance positions for their shots, with the effect that their eyes are nowhere near level. As discussed earlier, there will almost always be a subtle tilt to the head and eyes, and it's mostly likely more important, for your eyes to be in nearly the same position, relative to your body, than it is to try to imitate some perfect image of a pro player, that you like. I use some first grade singing, to teach something about the compromising positions, in which we put our eyes.

'The eye bone is connected to the head bone. The head bone is connected to the body bone,' is something I say to show players, that they move their heads too much. Those excessive motions of the eyes, are created by the way they move their body, in the final stages of seeing the ball, compromising their vision.

In case you didn't know, you will actually need to go off balance, in order to run, but even in that off balance running, maintaining relatively still eyes and head aid in tracking. The most critical thing to do is using the dynamic balance of going from the off balance moving, coming to a nearly ideal balanced position with almost no head movement. I say almost none, because some people are prone to try so hard to keep their heads perfectly still, that they create extra upper body tension, and that doesn't help much either.

Players also tilt their heads in odd ways, and have other strange head motions, that seem to be born from an idea, trying to keep their eye on the ball, by turning their head. Coaches regularly see players moving their head forward before contact, we also see players who think they are doing well to get ready for a shot, especially a volley.

Players have been taught to be disciplined, by constantly bouncing up and down, to be ready to spring for the ball, as though it's a good thing to do.

Being very active is taught as a positive footwork training. Unfortunately, bouncing up and down, actually works to compromise the vision of the ball, meaning that there will be two objects in motion, the ball and your eyes. Requiring constant movement, creates a confusing environment, by asking players to do something that compromises their vision.

## The Still Moments

Being relatively still, although not completely stopped, at the moment of the opponent's contact with the ball, can reduce the combined motion of ball, racquet and person by 50 to 100%. Also, our eyes require relative stillness in order to able to focus. Even while tracking, reconciling the arc of the ball is easier, if your head is not moving up and down, changing the eyes position to the relative movement of the ball. If then, the player can move efficiently with a minimum of bouncing their eyes around, they can track the ball much better in flight. Take note at how smoothly top players move, and how that makes for the best possible conditions for vision.

When you watch the top players, look carefully for how hard they fight to get in position, so that they will have a 'still moment' prior to striking the ball. Federer will always be the greatest example of this. When you have almost no lower body movement for a brief moment, your eyes can focus better. As a point of special emphasis, it bears repeating, that it does not mean to stop, do not come to a complete stop, instead relatively still ,to allow for you to move away immediately after completion of the shot. When you come to a complete stop, you create inertia, which makes it much more difficult to get moving again.

Johnny Bench, perhaps the greatest catcher in the history of baseball, and a huge tennis fan, recently compared returning a serve with hitting a fastball in baseball, that given the speeds and distances that those two skills are equally difficult. Johnny marveled at how returning a serve can be more difficult because the ball interacts with the ground, and the spin of the serve creates the need for a last minute adjustment.

**Therefore, it is imperative to see the ball at the bounce.**

Every time you can get in position, prior to the bounce for a still moment, that can be at least a neutral, and likely a very positive experience. Every time your opponent puts you out of position enough, that you are still on the move when the ball is bouncing, it's important to recognize that it's not an ideal visual moment and you are under pressure, so it's a great idea to track the ball well.

Fifty-Five

# Why Is It Important To Have An Origin Story?

*Just walk a mile in his moccasins
Before you abuse, criticize and accuse.
If just for one hour, you could find a way
To see through his eyes, instead of your own muse.
~ Mary T. Lathrap*

A fundamental understanding gained, in doing the research, into the true nature of the visual experience, is that everyone is different. As we get to the end of this study of visual training, it may be helpful for you and your students to read my own experience. When I was young, I was not such a great athlete, in any sport that required tracking a ball, or hitting a target. I was fast and aggressive but that was about it.

**My ability to find an object in space was very poor, which meant I had a hard time in athletics as a kid.**

I had an erratic ability to catch a ball, I could make very difficult catches, but quite often following the advice of my coaches, keeping my eye on the ball, I would drop the easiest ones. I told myself that I was just not good at catching anything. Of course, my father, grandfathers and all my coaches had seemingly told me around 10,000 times 'keep your eye on the ball'. I always thought I was trying to do that, and to be told the same thing, over and over again, did not build my confidence. It never seemed to help. What I was doing, did not match up with what they were saying.

Compounding my problem, I was deemed by school specialists to be 'hyperactive,' before ADD and ADHD became commonly diagnosed, and was put on heavy doses of Methylphenidate also known as Ritalin in those days, and now prescribed under many different brand names. That drug left me delirious, and doctors couldn't seem to get the dosage right, so I was left alone. I'm actually happy, not to have been medicated long term. Which leads me to the real 'why,' the main motivation of this book, is to help cure the vital piece that I needed to fix in order to become a decent tennis player?

**As I began to piece together enough information, over the years, I was able to become one of the better 5.0 level players in Northern California, and for me that was quite an accomplishment, since I felt I had a lot to overcome.**

I want to help people overcome the difficulty of poor performances. Many players play with a lack of confidence, dreading the moment that they lose the ball, and make the critical mistake. This happens with players, because coaches lack tools that actually work. 'Watch the ball' or 'keep your eye' on the ball are like using a hammer to try to turn a screw.

The internal pressure I felt, to try to do what all of my mentors wanted me to do, drove me to do, what I believe many of you out there do, which is to try too hard. I believe that my fight was overcompensating. By trying so hard to focus on the ball at all times, I made it harder to track the ball. The vast number of botched repetitions created an environment that led to an incredible amount of anxiety, frustration and anger, from myself and others, directed at me when I failed to make a play, dropped a ball, etc. Even through my teens and into my adult life, I would play out of the fear that I knew on a big shot, I might all of a sudden lose my concentration and miss the shot that I really need to hit in order to win the game. Maybe you can relate to this experience, and if one person can, then it's worth it to tell my own struggles.

**When I first began studying tennis coaching, in the early 90s, I had my first exposure to Ken DeHart, who was one of the few teaching anything about visual skills, that could be used on the tennis court.**

Over the years, I have continued to study, and as previously stated, after 28 years of teaching and learning, I thought I knew some things about vision, enough to write a book, but in doing the research for the book, I learned more than 100% more! Compared to the original edition, this fourth edition contains again more than 100% more content. So, bottom line we all need to have more empathy for the player who struggles, and they don't know why. I quit tennis 10 times out of frustration, only to keep coming back, now it seems like destiny. Sadly, many people will quit one time, and never come back.

### Breakthroughs Can Happen Later

When I first started coaching tennis, I was probably a 3.5 player, but in the matter of about 5 years I became a 4.5 and then one of the best 5.0 level players in NorCal especially in doubles where visual skills, and fast reflexes are even more valuable. For a few golden weeks, I felt like I was playing at a 5.5/6.0 level, because I was playing those people evenly, and seemingly no 4.5 player could stay on the court with me, before I fell back down to earth, but that's another story. Most of that education has come from The Inner Game of Tennis both books, including Inner Tennis: Playing The Game which I find to be more practical than the original book.

**Over the years I had multitude of trainings with great tennis professionals, among them, Ken DeHart, Jack Broudy, Don Henson, and Steve Stefanki, who have delved into the mind/body connection as it directly relates to visual acuity. Their influences and those of many others are found in this work.**

As I continued to progress, I became the guy who could make the winning shot in basketball, hit the passing shot on match point, get a two out hit, or a vital defensive play on a baseball diamond. May accuracy of shot, and reliable catching, has made me a sought after teammate. I overcame my personal demons, and no one I was playing with, knew that I had formerly been a sports failure. While none of that was achieved in a professional arena, it became my own personal triumph knowing, that I had overcome Attention Deficit Hyperactivity Disorder, and the attending issues that come with it, to where I am today. I do not think it's accurate that I am THE expert in this field, as some have suggested, I simply went about the business of collecting as much usable information as I could find, there are thousands of researchers more knowledgeable than me, but they didn't write this book.

It would not be such a stretch to say that the connection of mind/body connection training with the visual training, has helped me in my ability to read and write at a high level, and so the whole quality of my life has been improved. People make excuses for poor performance, by citing that they are ADD, or ADHD, and while much of that is very serious, what most people mean is that they lack discipline or do not know which skills to practice. Today, when I tell my students that I had been ADHD, they can't believe it, they think I am joking in a low key sarcastic way. Some of the strategies in this book have been the keys to help me to learn to focus well enough to be able to write multiple books, which I began to do in 2013.

**I was able to let go of the internal dialogue connected to 'watching the ball' as a subconscious command. I no longer have to overcompensate for something that's missing.**

The shift toward simply being aware of the ball and allowing my eyes to do what they can do naturally, if I get out of the way of my brain, brought a lot of joy and enjoyment of the sport, and has allowed me to unlock this for thousands of tennis players and some people in other sports. Now, I just have fun playing.

Fifty-Six

## How Bizarre Visual Events Can Create Empathy

*Empathy - The ability to understand
and share the feelings of another.
~ Oxford English Dictionary*

### My 'Major' Visual Incident

While in the midst of finishing the second edition of this book, I took a road trip to Los Angeles,  while driving home at night, I was having some very bad vision problems. I was seeing dark shapes, moving in front of the car, and other distracting and unnerving problems of perception. I felt like something was wrong with my eyes, or I was losing my mind, seeing things that were not really present. It seemed like there were animals crossing the road, but as I got closer, nothing was there. I saw a space, where I could no longer see the lines or reflectors in the road, and it was darker than dark, which made me automatically want to hit the brakes of my car. My eyes became very tired as I as driving, so I had to make numerous stops to rest. I began to worry that I had a torn retina, or one of the other myriad problems that can occur, from many years in the sun. At my appointment with an eye doctor it was discovered that... I need glasses. That's all, just glasses, and my prescription wasn't incredibly strong.

**In retrospect, I came to the realization that I had probably needed glasses for years.**

Not only do I now have driving glasses for distance, but I also use reading glasses that help with my astigmatism, which I did not know I had. I now can see the logo on the ball again, and leaves on trees. When I first received my glasses, I also understood for the first time why they call it HD TV.  I can drive much longer without getting tired and my players don't question my calls. In fact, one amusing part of my story is that I was coaching juniors, and I thought I saw a player make a bad call, so I questioned it, only to have both players say it was a good call, looking at me curiously. I had to apologize a couple times, and learn not to intrude. I really never thought I would be so happy to have glasses. Maybe it's time for you to go to the eye doctor, making sure that you let your doctor know that you play tennis and need to be able to see well from 3 to 80 feet away.  Also, be sure to have empathy for those who might not see the ball as well as you might expect.

## Labeling a Junior Player: Cheater

I was running a tournament, and a young boy was making plenty of 'mistakes' on his calls. The opponent was perplexed, but did not call for a lines person, but I made myself available, to be ready, in case he wanted one. The thing that struck me about the boy, who was 'cheating,' was that he seemed not to have any guile. He was pleasant, and he didn't shrink back or avoid eye contact from the crowd after a bad call, which real cheaters often do. Real cheaters have a presence about them.

**Then I began watching the boy's father, who seemed to cringe every time his son called a close ball out**.

I counted at least 8 calls that were incorrect. I think the dad was perplexed at why that was happening, but didn't know what to do. After the match I called them both together, and told them this: 'Sir, I think you are a great dad, and your son seems like a very nice young boy. I also thought I saw you looking uncomfortable, when your son made what looked like mistakes on a few calls, and yes there were mistakes made. I wouldn't call him a cheater. Can you do me a favor and promise to take him to the eye doctor at the earliest possible time? I am guessing that he isn't seeing as well as he could.' The father was a little confused, as tournament people aren't supposed to be proactive and actually care about children. They went away, after not saying much, but we had agreed that there were bad calls.

A few months later, at another tournament the father came running my way, and the way he was running, had me worried that I should protect myself. I was ready. Before he got 10 feet away I heard him saying, 'Thank you, thank you, thank you! We went to the eye doctor, my son now plays with contact lens in place, and HE IS PLAYING SO MUCH BETTER!' So, that was a relief, and we miss opportunities to work with people to help solve problems, instead of stigmatizing them as 'cheater'.

## Two Feet In

Another match I saw, a player called a ball out that was fully two feet inside the line. His opponent went a little crazy, and said, "NO WAY, that ball was two feet in!". He went to the opponent's side of the court, which you are not supposed to do, to point at the spot where it landed. The player who made the bad call, pointed to a place, exactly two feet out, on the other side of the line. The concerned player, realizing that perhaps his opponent is dyslexic, went to get a lines-person. Two calls were overturned, but the match proceeded without any negativity because the problem was solved. It wasn't anything personal, the issue was simply that the opponent had a visual issue.

This is most likely the cause of a very high percentage of bad calls.

Of course, there are those who will make bad calls on purpose on big points to win by really cheating, but those people and calls are really in the minority. In many years of running tournaments, I found that about 80% of errors are just because making a call is not easy, and mistakes are made among those, a large percentage could be because people could be helped by corrective lenses. About 15% of errors are due to the psychological blindness of the person, who wished the ball to be out, so they called it out. It's as though their brain convinced them it was what they wanted to see. This kind of 'cheating' can be brought on by tremendous parental and coaching pressure to win. About 5%, or one in twenty are criminal calls, where the opponent knowing that it's break point or game point, they are going to call a ball on the line out, because their coach or their parent expects them to do so, or they have made up their mind that this is what they need to do preemptively, before the other player does it to them.

### Conclusions: Don't Jump To Them

When you are playing, and there is an initial bad call, study your opponent. Look at them, look at the line, see what they do. If they are attentive, they will notice your body language. They might reverse their call. If they do, you can trust them, making a new friend. If they don't, maybe you are wrong. They are closer. If you are sure they made a mistake, chalk it up to bad eyesight. On the second bad call, say their name: "Eric, are you sure?" adding the name removes the anonymity factor, if they chirp back that they are sure, then either they really can't see, or they are cheating. On the third bad call get a lines-person, because they simply don't see well enough to play fair, they need help. If you take it from that perspective of their visual inadequacy, it saves you from making the calling a lines person as a personal attack.

Fifty-Seven

## What Should I Eat For Eye Health? Which Foods To Eat For Development, Improvement and Maintainence Of Vision

*Eat your foods as your medicines, or you will
have to eat your medicines as your foods.
~ Unknown, possibly Hippocrates*

The quote above is believed to possibly, have been attributed to Hippocrates the father of medicine, but many medical experts use this same statement as their own. If you are like me, then you grew up with the idea that you should eat carrots and other great sources of Vitamin A / Betacarotene, for better eye sight. I have good news and bad news.

The good news is that there are a lot more nutrients beyond simple vitamins, that are known to be supportive of eye development, healthy, and disease prevention.

Some foods will help in the developmental stages, others in your present ability to have visual acuity, and still others for your long term eye health, for seeing well into old age. The bad news is that you most likely will need to eat your vegetables, and add more 'green stuff' to your diet. You will want more than just carrots. If you are a vegan, you might find it difficult to get a complete range of nutrients for your eyes, in high enough concentrations, so I hope this information helps guide your thinking.

According to Dr. James McDonnell, a pediatric ophthalmologist at Loyola University Health System in Maywood, Ill., "Make a colorful plate, especially the greens, blues and reds. Certain foods have distinct benefits to the eyes in addition to overall health, including many of the trendy superfoods such a kale, broccoli and sweet potatoes." As you will see in the lists below, that different kinds of seafood are among the richest sources of nutritional benefit to developing, performing and aging eyes.

This chapter is not meant to be exhaustive, so do your own research, but when you make your shopping list, you can look for all of these beneficial foods. Bless your children, and aging parents with a great diet so that they will develop with their best vision, and see longer and better throughout their lifespan.

**The Shopping List -** These nine nutrients cover much of what you can eat to help you build, fuel and maintain your eyes.

***Water - well, ok it's not a nutrient, but*** being very well hydrated is important for your overall health, but also critical to the wellness of your eyes. I now use a fitness tracker that pairs with a scale that measures many things including my overall hydration. In one month I improved my overall water percentage by 1.7% and it has made an amazing difference with my health, and my eyes! Caution: You might be shocked to find out that you are not as hydrated as you thought you might be.

***Astaxanthin*** - helps from developing cataracts, macular degeneration and blindness.

Seaweed and Wild Salmon (not farmed) are excellent choices high in Astaxanthin.
- Salmon or Seaweed
- Shrimp
- Crab
- Lobster
- Red Trout
- Krill

***Omega 3*** "Studies show that individuals who ate oily fish such as tuna, sardines, herring and salmon at least once a week were 50 percent less likely to develop neovascular [wet] macular degeneration than those who ate fish less than once per week," McDonnell said.

What are the best sources of omega-3?

Fish sources
Vegan sources
Supplements

There are three main types of omega-3 fatty acid, which are called ALA, DHA, and EPA.

Plant sources, such as nuts and seeds, are rich in ALA, while fish, seaweed, and algae can provide DHA and EPA fatty acids. Eating a variety of omega-3 sources is important.

For each fish below, the serving size is 3 ounces (oz):

1. Mackerel - 0.59 g DHA, 0.43 g EPA
2. Salmon - 1.24 g DHA, 0.59 g EPA
3. Sea-bass - 0.47 g DHA, 0.18 g EPA
4. Oysters - 0.14 ALA, 0.23 g DHA, 0.30 g EPA

5. Sardines - 0.74 g DHA. 0.45 g EPA
6. Shrimp - 0.12 g DHA, 0.12 g EPA
7. Trout - 0.44 g DHA, 0.40 g EPA
8. Seaweed and algae — amounts vary widely

Seaweed, nori, spirulina, and chlorella are one of the few plant groups that contain DHA and EPA.

9. Chia seeds - 5.055 g ALA per 1-oz serving.
10. Hemp seeds - 2.605 g ALA 3 tablespoons
11. Flaxseeds - 6.703 g ALA per tablespoon.
12. Walnuts - 3.346 g ALA per cup.
13. Edamame - 0.28 g ALA per half cup
14. Kidney beans - 0.10 g ALA per half-cup.
15. Soybean oil - 0.923 g ALA per tablespoon

## *Anthocyanins*

"Blueberries, bilberries and especially black currants contain high amounts of anthocyanins and help to maintain the health of the cornea and blood vessels in every part of the eye," McDonnell said. "They also help reduce the risk of cataracts and macular degeneration as well as decrease inflammatory eye disease and diabetic retinopathy."

Black raspberries
Black currants
Blueberries
Blackberries
Red cabbage
Black plums
Red radish
Red raspberries

## *Vitamin D*

Vitamin D helps prevent age-related macular degeneration and improve vision.
~ Oscar F. Chuyn

"Safe sun exposure, fish oils, fatty fish and, to a lesser extent, beef liver, cheese, egg yolks and certain mushrooms contain this master hormone, which acts on more than 4,000 genes," McDonnell said. He added that vitamin D3 supplementation has been shown to help prevent age-related macular degeneration, reduce retinal inflammation and improve vision.

Primary Sources
Sunlight
Tuna
Mackerel

Salmon
Foods fortified with vitamin D
Secondary Sources
Beef liver
Cheese
Egg yolks

## *Zeaxanthin*

Greens such as...

Kale
Spinach
Romaine lettuce

...pack a nutrient called zeaxanthin. This nutrient, which McDonnell said reduces the risk of age-related macular degeneration, is found in dark green vegetables such as kale, broccoli, collards, raw spinach and romaine lettuce. "Lightly cooking these vegetables increases your body's ability to absorb these nutrients," McDonnell said.

## *Lutein*

"The best source is from organic eggs laid by pastured organic hens. You can also take supplements made from marigold flowers," McDonnell said.

## *Lutein and Zeaxanthin Combined*

Dark Leafy Greens
Peas
Summer Squash
Pumpkin
Brussels Sprouts
Broccoli
Asparagus
Lettuce
Carrots
Pistachios
Marigold Flower Supplement

## *Bioflavonoids*

Citrus fruits
Cherries
Tea
Red Wine
Broccoli

Red and Yellow Onions

You can find bioflavonoids in the pulp and white core that runs through the center of citrus fruits, green peppers, lemons, limes, oranges, cherries, and grapes. Quercitin is a highly concentrated form of bioflavonoids found in broccoli, citrus fruits, and red and yellow onions. Foods high in bioflavonoids may help you stay healthy. Hosts of experiments on bioflavonoids have suggested that these key nutrients help increase immune system activation. These biochemically active substances accompany vitamin C in plants and act as an antioxidant.

## *Beta-carotene*

Beta-carotene, contained in carrots, sweet potatoes, spinach, kale and butternut squash, protects you against night blindness and dry eyes, the eye doctor noted. It's easy to get enough Beta-carotene through the following foods, so supplementation is not necessary and can be harmful if taken too often.

The foods highest in beta carotene include:

dark leafy greens — kale and spinach
sweet potatoes
carrots
broccoli
butternut squash
cantaloupe
red and yellow peppers
apricots
broccoli
peas
romaine lettuce
paprika
cayenne
chili
parsley
cilantro
marjoram
sage
coriander

My recommendation is to add 1 item from every nutrient group. Keep in mind that the items high on the list are better sources, so go as high on the list as you can. Be sure to mix things up, trying some new foods, herbs and spices to keep it interesting.

Fifty-Eight

## A Healthy Mind In A Healthy Body

*The best day to plant a tree is 20 years ago,
the next best day is today.*
*~ Confucius*

In this chapter, let's go outside the realm of pure sports performance to reach into general health and well-being, which can also have a dramatic effect on performance. Let's look at developmental issues through the lens of overcoming perceived 'deficits', and also through that of parenting a child. Ultimately, letting go of any shame for the conditions we are born into is helpful, and simply observe what is your current state, or the state of your child, then seek courses of action to develop in that area. This book has already shown that everyone has their own particular unique visual issue, so you are not alone simply because yours comes with a diagnosis.

The eye is literally an extension of the brain. It is estimated that over 60% of the brain has some duties associated with vision input. Compared to the sense of touch (8%) and hearing (3%), the eyes are the by far the dominant input devices for the brain. Because of this, any condition that hampers vision or the processing of vision may result in problems learning. These conditions are not only varied but also range from mild to severe. When diagnosed and treated early, people have a better chance of learning efficiently.

### Risk Factors Of Visual Learning Issues

Heredity can be a large risk factor in all types of learning and vision problems. Having a family history of learning or vision problems puts you at a greater risk. After conception, during development in the womb, the baby can be exposed to many positive and negative influences. Negative influences include the mental/emotional state of the mother, diet, and poor lifestyle choices including tobacco, alcohol, and both legal and illegal drug use. Let's assume that you are an active healthy person, that's great.

**If you are coming out of less than healthy environments, then it's worth taking note of ways to address what you are leaving, to enter a fully healthy state.**

After birth, conditions that are negative to healthy development such as neglect, abuse or a stress-filled home environment can also lead to developmental delays in many areas. To give yourself and your child the best chance at success, nurture him or her from the beginning. Reading to your child in the womb is one of the best things you can do. If you have been raised in difficult circumstances, moving to a more positive mindset and doing a deep dive into detoxification, fitness and great nutrition could help you turn the corner with performance.

## Symptoms

A good doctor should be testing the child from birth through the first years of life for important learning and developmental milestones. After entering school, children may be tested for a learning problem, if certain symptoms or history is concerning. There is a balance between offering extra support to your struggling student at home, and having them labeled by the school district.

**Once a label is applied, it is rarely removed.**

With my son, he was not reading in first grade like the others, and it was recommended that he join a 'pull out' program. After careful thought and consideration, my wife and I decided against that, and worked with my son on his reading. By the end of second grade, he was performing at a high level, and he became an outstanding writer. At the age of 23, he is the one who edited my book The Athlete Centered Coach.

At earlier ages developmental delays such as crawling, walking, talking, and general behavior based on norms. Vision problems could result in symptoms such as squinting to see up close or far away, closing or covering one eye, tilting of the head, rubbing the eyes, red and/or watery eyes, headaches, unusual fatigue while performing vision-related tasks such as reading, writing, coloring, or watching digital devices.

**While these symptoms are relatively easy to observe, symptoms of visual processing can be much harder to detect.**

Many conditions may be difficult to test at extremely young ages, but observant parents, caregivers, and teachers can observe subtle behaviors and not so subtle behaviors that would be symptoms of learning problems that may be associated with the visual system. These include reversal of letters and words beyond the age of seven, poor reading ability and comprehension, lack of interest in schoolwork, especially reading tasks, and disruptive behavior in the classroom and outside the classroom.

## Diagnosis

A comprehensive eye exam is the first step to determine if visual problems are contributing to learning problems. Simply correcting uncorrected refractive error such as near or farsighted and astigmatism can solve many problems quickly and easily. Other conditions such as the inability for the eyes to work comfortably together (binocular vision) and focus properly (accommodation) are also tested during an eye exam. Testing for amblyopia, sometimes called lazy eye will also be performed. Some doctors of optometry who specialize in vision-related learning problems may have a more extensive battery of tests that often include pencil/paper tasks, visual memory testing, and perceptual testing such as copying forms and reading efficiency testing. I once had a young student, whose eyes did not track together.

**There was no mention of this with the parents, and my opinion is that she made more errors and had slightly skewed perception of the incoming ball.**

After developing a close and trusting relationship with the parents, one day I told them that I thought it wise for them to see an optometrist about her eye tracking issue where both eyes did not look straight ahead at the same time. They did go to the doctor who prescribed some eye exercises and her eyes straightened out. This can be a very sensitive subject and must be handled with extreme care and professionalism.

### Treatment

After a diagnosis is made, treatment must be initiated immediately in order to prevent further consequences, primarily falling behind in school. It's obvious that in order to promote the greatest possible learning in childhood, that early diagnosis and treatment are most helpful. As we get older addressing these issues is still possible, but can be a bit more difficult. As I discussed earlier, I believe my astigmatism made it very difficult for me academically, and the writing of my first book was a very difficult chore.

The treatment may be as simple as full time or part-time use of corrective lenses. It may also be as complex as a team of professionals providing multiple learning activities. An IEP or individual education plan, through your school, may be implemented to guide the child, so that he/she is not overwhelmed in the classroom.

Physical therapists or occupational therapists, along with doctors of optometry, vision therapists, may also be brought in for treatment and progress testing.

As Dr. Cherylle Calder states, many varied visual experiences can also help, like climbing, doing gymnastics, or other challenging visual tasks. Out of school learning activities such as children's museums, library visits, and even simply being read to can also help young learners find fun ways to learn.

## Prevention

As with any condition, early detection and treatment is desired. This action will ensure the young learner with problems is given an opportunity to become the best he/she can be. For the purposes of this work, my main focus is the future sports performance, but that obviously takes a backseat to your academic future.

**Everything an infant observes, is a learning experience.**

Even if a child does not yet speak, he/she loves to hear voices and see colorful pictures and objects. Explaining things you do, or reciting nursery rhymes and singing simple songs will stimulate their young brains to continually seek to know more. You can play little games with balls, touching hands, or picking out small objects to develop visual acuity.

Fifty-Nine

# Maintain Healthy Eyes
# Early Warning Systems

Please read the next few chapters with caution. One tricky psychological phenomenon behind studying illness, is that many people are prone to think that they have an illness, which they do not. I am including some maladies in the book, simply so that you can be watchful, and take early action by seeing a doctor if needed. Your first step would always be to set yourself up to eliminate eye strain, Computer Vision Syndrome, make sure you are hydrated, and eating some of the foods that are great for your eyes.

### Acanthamoeba

Acanthamoeba is one of the most common organisms in the environment. Although, it rarely causes infection, when it does occur, it can threaten your vision.

Irritated eye — eye infection — keratitis. Recently, there have been increased reports of Acanthamoeba keratitis. The best defense against this infection is cleaning contact lenses properly. People without contact lenses are far less likely to encounter this malady.

### Causes & risk factors

Using tap water to clean and disinfect contact lenses, including the lens case.
Swimming with contact lenses, especially in freshwater lakes and rivers.
Acanthamoeba keratitis has been found in almost all water sources from pools to hot tubs and showers. Failure to follow contact lens care instructions could lead to infection.

### Symptoms

A red, frequently painful eye infection that doesn't improve with traditional treatment.

Feeling of something in the eye, excessive tearing, light sensitivity, and blurred vision.

Red, irritated eyes that last for an unusually long time after removing your contact lenses.

## Diagnosis

The best course of action is to see a doctor of optometry with symptoms. Do not hesitate to tell your doctor of improper contact lens or case care, as accurate information can lead to a precise diagnosis and proper treatment.

Doctors will use the patient's history, symptoms and lens-care habits to determine if the patient has Keratitis. Pain is typically out of proportion to signs. The doctor will perform a complete eye health examination and may order lab tests or consider a biopsy.

## Treatment

Topical agents applied to the infected area over months.
Removal of damaged tissues.
The doctor may consider a biopsy if the condition worsens.

## Prevention

Always wash hands before handling contact lenses.
Rub and rinse the surface of the contact lens before storing.
Use only sterile products recommended by your doctor of optometry to clean and disinfect your lenses. Saline solution and rewetting drops are not designed to disinfect lenses.
Avoid using tap water to wash or store contact lenses.
Contact lens solution must be discarded upon opening the case, and fresh solution used each time the contact lens is placed in the case.
Replace lenses using your doctor's prescribed schedule.
Do not sleep in contact lenses unless prescribed by your doctor and never after swimming.
Never swap lenses with someone else.
Never put contact lenses in your mouth or use saliva to wet the contact lens.
See your doctor of optometry regularly for contact lens evaluation.
If you experience RSVP (redness, secretions, visual blurring or pain), return to your doctor of optometry immediately.

# Anterior Uveitis

Anterior uveitis is an inflammation of the middle layer of the eye. This middle layer includes the iris (colored part of the eye) and adjacent tissue, known as the ciliary body.

## Irritated Eyes

## Causes And Risk Factors

Anterior uveitis can result from a trauma to the eye, such as being hit in the eye or having a foreign body in the eye. It can also be associated with general health problems such as rheumatoid arthritis, syphilis, tuberculosis, sarcoid, viral (herpes simplex, herpes zoster, cytomegalovirus) or no obvious underlying cause.

## Symptoms

Red, sore and inflamed eye
Blurred vision
Sensitivity to light
Small, or irregular-shaped pupil

## Diagnosis

The symptoms of anterior uveitis can be similar to those of other eye conditions. Therefore, a doctor of optometry will carefully examine the front and inside of the eye with a unique microscope using high magnification. A doctor of optometry may also perform or arrange for other diagnostic tests to help pinpoint the cause.

## Treatment

Prescription eye drops, which dilate the pupils, in combination with anti-inflammatory drugs. Dilating drops will blur vision and increase light sensitivity. However, by relaxing the iris muscles, the eye will be much more comfortable. The treatment takes several days or—in some cases—several weeks. Never discontinue medications early as this could result in a rapid reoccurrence of the uveitis. If the condition does not respond well to prescription drops, injections of steroid medications just under the outer tissue of the eye may be needed. Occasionally, oral steroid medications will be used.

## Prevention

Anterior uveitis in an otherwise healthy individual cannot be prevented since often the cause is not known. However, in persons with auto-immune diseases, taking care of those conditions can lead to better health for the body, including the eyes. To prevent serious complications, including permanent loss of some or all vision, early diagnosis and proper treatment is essential.

If untreated, glaucoma, cataract or retinal edema can develop and cause permanent loss of vision. Anterior Uveitis has also been called Iritis. Anterior Uveitis usually responds well to treatment; however, the condition tends to recur.

# Accommodative Dysfunction

Accommodative dysfunction is an eye-focusing problem resulting in blurred vision, up close and/or far away. It is frequently found in children or adults who have extended near-work demand. This is different from Computer Vision Syndrome, in that it affects the ability to focus at different depths off field, and track approaching objects.

## Causes and Risk Factors

The cause seems to be the inability to use the two eyes in proper binocular vision function

Visual demands increasing in their work

Unable to focus from prolonged near centered tasks, without interventions

## Symptoms

Inability to change focus from near too far without blurring

Transient blurred vision

Abnormal postural adaptations (too close or too far away / working distance)

Visual stress, headaches, decreased comprehension of material

Inconsistent work productivity, diminished accuracy

Avoidance of visually demanding tasks

Distractibility-inconsistent, inaccurate visual attention, concentration or awareness

Fatigue, eye movement, illusory perceptions

## Diagnosis

Comprehensive Eye health and vision examination

Patient History – complaints/symptoms

Binocular evaluation of sustenance visual abilities

## Treatment

Improve sustenance visual abilities/processing to look from near to far-Optometric Vision therapy/Vision Enhancement procedures with lenses and prisms-treatments in and out of the office.

Glasses or Contact lenses to correct an undetected refractive error-(two Rx's may be necessary for one pair of glasses or CLs-antifatigue RX)

# Amblyopia - Lazy Eye

Lazy Eye is often associated with crossed eyes, or is a large difference in the degree of nearsightedness or farsightedness between the two eyes. It usually develops before age 6 and does not affect side vision. Eyeglasses or contact lenses cannot fully correct the reduced vision caused by amblyopia if vision was not developed within the critical period.

## Causes And Risk Factors

Missing comprehensive eye exams at 6 months of age AND 3 years of age.
A high prescription that has gone uncorrected with glasses or contacts
Family history
Premature birth
Developmentally disabled
Eye turn — strabismus, one eye turned out or inward from center
Visual deprivation congenital cataract, ptosis and/or corneal opacities
Large refractive errors

## Symptoms

Symptoms may include noticeably favoring one eye or a tendency to bump into objects on one side.
Symptoms are not always obvious.

## Diagnosis

Early diagnosis increases the chance of a complete recovery.

The American Optometric Association recommends that children have a comprehensive optometric examination by 6 months of age and again at age 3. Lazy eye will not go away on its own. If left undiagnosed until the preteen, teen or adult years, treatment takes longer and is often less effective.

## Treatment

Treatment for lazy eye may include a combination of prescription lenses, prisms, vision therapy and eye patching.
In vision therapy, patients learn how to use the two eyes together, which helps prevent lazy eye from reoccurring.

Sixty

## How To Avoid Computer Vision Syndrome (Part One)

*The graphics are better outside.*
*~ BP*

The more you use a computer, or other electronic device, the more likely you are to develop some serious negative patterns of vision, posture and balance. If you are also going to be a competitive tennis player, then you really must follow these guidelines outlined below, or do even more than what is minimally recommended. When I am writing a book, I never sit at my computer for more than 30 minutes, and I have everything on my screen set up to be ideal for my eyes, using dark backgrounds and white font, using the color blindness settings, fonts etc.

**You need to know the symptoms, causes and risks of overworking your eyes on a screen very close to your face for extended periods.**

You will find that there are quite a few things you can do to take charge of this so that you will have better overall vision longer in life, and maintain your ability to compete in tennis at a high level. With so many people working from home nowadays, it's vital that you set up your work space in a way that allows you to be optimally positioned and allows you to get up and out.

### The Form Of What You Read

A good source on reading research tells me that Verdana is the font that leads to the best reading and comprehension for most people. Since I switched to Verdana for all emails, writing and everything I read on a computer, I find that to be true for me. Using Verdana as a guide for simplicity, maybe you will find a similar font that you like better. For reading pages in print on computer paper or a book Garamond was found to be best. Many computers do not offer this font, and my simple work around is to use Georgia or Geneva.

**I use Georgia and Geneva exclusively in my books.**

Geneva for titles, and Georgia for the body of text. According to the research, sans serif fonts present better to your eye on a computer, and serif fonts with the little detailed edges are better for your eye to latch onto in print. It's obvious that when you use these settings and make comprehension easier for yourself and others, then your work will be easier and more effective and you will not have to spend as long at the computer.

## Manage Your Computer Time

The average American worker spends seven hours a day on the computer. At the very minimum you should use the 20/20/20 Rule, which means that every 20 minutes you should look at something more than 20 feet away for twenty full seconds. It's much better if you can get up, walk around and give your full attention to numerous objects at varying depth. You can also perform some of the eye exercises in other chapters.

**Wearable tech is helpful here, where you can set it up to remind you to get up and walk around.**

Use your phone or other device to set alerts and notifications to get up and move. Late in 2020 I started in the world of fitness trackers, and found that I really enjoy the gamification of doing these things for my health and vision.

## Causes And Risk Factors

Viewing a computer or digital screen makes your eyes work harder. There are vision related syndromes that commonly occur when you spend too long at a screen. The longer you continuing in the pattern of staying too long with your screen, no matter what kind of screen it is, the greater likelihood of developing Computer Vision Syndrome (CVS).

**Viewing a computer or digital screen is different from reading a printed page.**

The letters on the computer or device are not as precise as printed words, the contrast is not as great and the presence of glare and reflections on the screen may make viewing difficult.

Commonly the viewing angle for reading on a screen is different from that of a book, although a handheld device may mimic that of printed words. The placement of the screen can create additional demands on your vision. In addition, the presence of even minor vision problems can often significantly affect comfort and performance at a computer or while using other digital screen devices. Uncorrected or under corrected vision problems can be major contributing factors to computer-related eyestrain.

**If you get glasses, make sure they have a blue light blocking film, and work closely with your doctor to get the distance of focus just**

**right.**

When I first had reading glasses the doctor used an average distance for focus, but I have long arms, and enjoy reading from further away than most people, so on the next go around we got that dialed in, and that helped my reading, which meant less eye strain. As I sit here typing this I am happy that my glasses are set up the way they are. Some people tilt their heads at odd angles, because their glasses aren't designed for looking at a computer, or they bend toward the screen in order to see it clearly. Their postures can result in muscle spasms or pain in the neck, shoulder or back, and those will not help your tennis game.

In most cases, symptoms of CVS occur because the visual demands of the task exceed the visual abilities of the individual to comfortably perform them. At greatest risk for developing CVS are those persons who spend two or more continuous hours at a computer or using a digital screen device every day.

### Symptoms Of CVS

Eyestrain
Headaches
Blurred vision
Dry eyes
Neck and shoulder pain

### These symptoms may be caused by:

Poor lighting.
Glare on a digital screen
Improper viewing distances
Poor seating posture
Uncorrected vision problems
A combination of these factors

I have a lamp near my desk to backlight myself and bring warmth to the lighting in my work space. I'm not sure if the monitor I am using is the lowest in glare, but I seem to be happy with the slightly matte appearance. On my iPad I use a screen protector that not only has a matte appearance which almost eliminates glare, but it also gives a texture that feels like paper for the stylus. You can find those for about $10 if you shop well.

Whether or not I have the best seating posture, one thing I do is change the height of my chair, so I go up and down, so that I am not always in the same position. I have a scheduled annual exam with my eye doctor and he does a great job of letting me know if I really need glasses, or if they are optional because my vision only changed a little bit. If you take some time to manage these issues, you can help maintain good performance or maybe even enhance your performance on court.

Sixty-One

# How To Avoid Computer Vision Syndrome (Part Two)

*That tree looks so realistic!*
*~ BP*

## Total Screen Time

The extent to which individuals experience visual symptoms often depends on the level of their visual abilities and the amount of time spent looking at a digital screen. I used to look at my computer often, my phone almost obsessively, and my iPad for certain projects with using apps unique to that platform. In order to reduce screen time, I have an established limit of how much time I will sit at the computer and it's not a long time, but I understand that your job might require you to sit at a computer for many hours.

**Take frequent breaks, even for under one minute.**

I also removed all social media and other distracting apps, from my phone, and my screen time there has diminished, to only essential communication. I am spending more time on my tablet, but that has a great matte screen protector. The matte finish cuts down on glare, even though the device itself features an anti-glare display, I find that matte is the best. The result is the most pleasant and accurate retina display available in my arsenal. The use of darker backgrounds on all devices has also been good to reduce glare and blue light, while also increasing battery life.

## Unresolved Eye Issues

Vision problems like farsightedness, astigmatism, inadequate eye focusing, eye coordination abilities, aging changes of the eyes, such as presbyopia, can all contribute to the development of visual symptoms when using a computer or digital screen device. I have an astigmatism which had gone undiagnosed for many years, and this made reading very difficult for me, but after getting glasses, it was night and day different.

## Stern Caution: Act Now!

Many of the visual symptoms experienced by users are only temporary and will decline after stopping computer work or use of the digital device. However, some individuals may experience continued reduced visual abilities, such as blurred distance vision, even after stopping work at a computer. If nothing is done to address the cause of the problem, the symptoms will continue to recur and perhaps worsen with future digital screen use. It's obvious that today is the day to start new habits in how you use your electronics.

## Computer Glasses For Those With Good Eye Sight

Players who do not require the use of eyeglasses for other daily activities may benefit from glasses designed specifically for computer use. Before I knew that I needed prescription glasses, I had begun experimenting with different types of computer glasses and settled on one pair that seemed most comfortable and blocked the most blue light.

Eyeglasses or contact lenses prescribed for general use may not be adequate for computer work. Lenses prescribed to meet the unique visual demands of computer viewing may be needed. Special lens designs, lens powers or lens tints or coatings may help to maximize visual abilities and comfort. Make sure your doctor knows exactly what you need, as unfortunately not every eye doctor is as good as mine, so be a good consumer.

## Work Your Eyes Out!

Some computer users experience problems with eye focusing or eye coordination that can't be adequately corrected with eyeglasses or contact lenses. A program of vision therapy may be needed to treat these specific problems. Try eyegym.com. Some of the exercises in this book can be considered eye therapy. Actively working to see things differently is the most important aspect to maintain a wider range of visual abilities. Eye exercises help remediate deficiencies in eye movement, eye focusing, and eye teaming and reinforce the eye-brain connection.

## How Should You Align Your Viewing Angle?

Most people find it more comfortable to view a computer when the eyes are looking slightly downward. Optimally, the computer screen should be 15 to 20 degrees below eye level (about 4 or 5 inches) as measured from the center of the screen and 20 to 28 inches from the eyes. Immediately after learning this piece of data, I was happy to discover that I had already set my up my desk to those specifications.

## Reading Material At Desk

These materials should be located above the keyboard and below the monitor. If this is not possible, a document holder can be used beside the monitor. The goal is to position the documents, so the head does not need to be repositioned from the document to the screen.

### Location of Screen

Position the computer screen to avoid glare, particularly from overhead lighting or windows. Use blinds or drapes on windows and replace the light bulbs in desk lamps with bulbs of lower wattage.

### Anti-Glare Screens

If there is no way to minimize glare from light sources, consider using a screen glare filter. These filters decrease the amount of light reflected from the screen. Some computers and lap tops feature matte screen finish, and I found that when I was using laptops that matte finish was highly desirable.

### Seating Position

Chairs should be comfortably padded and conform to the body. Chair height should be adjusted so the feet rest flat on the floor. Arms should be adjusted to provide support while typing and wrists shouldn't rest on the keyboard when typing.

### Rest Breaks

To prevent eyestrain, try to rest eyes when using the computer for long periods. Resting the eyes for 15 minutes after two hours of continuous computer use. Also, for every 20 minutes of computer viewing, look into the distance for 20 seconds to allow the eyes a chance to refocus. Those two items are what experts say is minimal. I try to never sit at the computer for more than 30 minutes before getting up and moving around, but that is also the desire to defeat a sedentary lifestyle. Generally, I have one or two bouts of writing for 30 minutes, then I do most of my work on my tablet, but might return to the desk for a few minutes at a time to return emails.

### Blinking On Purpose

To minimize the chances of developing dry eye when using a computer, try to blink frequently. Blinking keeps the front surface of the eye moist.

Take one action today to adjust your workspace to make it more eye friendly.

Sixty-Two

# Is There Social Proof Of These Principles? How Players Responded To Visual Issues, Learning To Win

One of the best results that has come from my time as a coach was when I began teaching everyone on my team visual skills, not only how to see the ball, but also how to hit targets on the court. In that league there was quite a bit of parity amongst the top players, and the league champion often had at least one loss during the season. Our league perennially had multiple participants in sectional play, but did not often make it out of the first round. In short order my team became a force at the sectional level, with two upset victories in the first year, defeating the #8, and #1 seeded teams before losing in the semifinals, but the next year coming in as the #3 seed, beat #2 and #1 in the same day in 97 degree heat, coming back from a 3-1 deficit in the final. Visual training played a major role in winning a sectional title without a single player ranked in the top 50.

## Stephen's Dramatic, But Simple Comeback

In our league singles final, my player Stephen was a bit out of sorts, and found himself quickly down 4-1 with two breaks against. His opponent was a known fast starter and a bit of a streaky player, capable of ending points quickly and stringing them together. The previous year Stephen was down to that player 6-1, and 4-0 in the second set before coming back to win. It seemed that every match between these two, it always looked really bad for our guy at the beginning. Again Stephen was down two breaks, so on the changeover the message was very simple. 'Pay attention to your contact point'.

**That was it.**

Simply bringing his awareness back to the most important moment in the game, where the ball and strings make impact. It's where the most important work gets done. If you do that well, it can make up for a lot of other idiosyncrasies. Stephen had looked like he was at sea, and had been fooled by well disguised spins, changes of pace and placements. Immediately after readjusting his objective, he cleaned up his game and within just a few minutes he came back quickly to 4-4. The crowd watching seemed to be impressed with how quickly that two break lead evaporated. Stephen only lost two more games the rest of the match, before winning 7-5, 6-1 asserting himself as the dominant two time champion of the league. There were no other technical or tactical adjustments made that day. Just a simple guide to fully experience the contact point on each ball, all you really need to do is look at that place for that to happen.

## Aaron's Dialing In Accuracy

Aaron was a sophomore when he started playing tennis, and was a very quiet young man. He did not have extremely impressive technique, as his strokes were very compact and seemed even a little tense. I was a coach with 42 kids on my team, and it was hard to pay attention to every match with 7 courts humming, especially with varsity. I managed to see most of Aaron's Junior Varsity match late in the season, noticing that he had a good concept for moving players around on the court to create openings, he obviously had developed his own ability to hit targets on the court. That summer we worked on his game a bit and the next year he made varsity.

The following summer we worked on refining the target area for his approach shots to an area that was about 40 sq. Ft., about 8 feet deep, by 5 feet wide in the backhand corner, and then he really only needed to make one volley to a target the same size in the deuce side near the 'Side T' at the service line.

Aaron's volleys were not great, but he was very solid at net if he didn't have to make two volleys. Using that ploy, the next year, he played #2 singles and went 15-1 on the season. Aaron then planned to play for his community college, and that would represent a significant jump up in competition from high school. He came from essentially nowhere, to become a college tennis player, simply by using his ability to hit targets on the court. The summer after his senior year we worked more and developed approach shots that went into a place that was only 4 feet deep and 5 feet wide in the backhand corner, and also the ability find an ideal position for a second volley, then to make his second volley a finishing shot, if the first volley did not win the point.

We did marginally improve Aaron's technique, but he still retained a fairly compact, and somewhat tense style that made him look beatable by opponent's, until they saw how good he was at hitting his spots on the court, moving them out of position, before he hit to the opening.

## Parent's Solve Child's Eye Pairing Issue

I had an 11 year old girl who came to a junior clinic that I was coaching and I immediately noticed that her left eye was slightly turned out from center. I had seen this before in students, waiting for a time when the parents felt comfortable with me that I could talk to them about going to a doctor about this condition. How it is that kids can make it to 11 without anyone noticing or intervening, I will never understand.

After a few months and some really good interactions with the parents, at the end of one clinic I asked if I could talk to the parents alone for a moment.

I simply pointed out that her eye is turned out slightly, and she has learned to adapt, it's not a deficit, although perhaps she might improve her vision somewhat if she undergoes eye therapy. Sure enough, the parents took that advice, went to the doctor and the girl went through a series of eye exercises to allow both eyes to track together. This girl who seemed at that time as though she might be able to join her high school team and participate, then improved dramatically in her tennis, and became the #2 player for her school. Speaking from pure vanity, it doesn't hurt your outward appearance when your eyes track straight forward.

## Rescuing Victory From The Jaws Of Meltdown Defeat

One of my girl players who I will not name was having a difficult time, she was having some personal issues, and her match looked fine with a 6-0 win in the first set and an early break in the second, but she began to coast, and her brother, who reminds her of her inner struggles, showed up to watch her. The other girl won two games in a row to make it even in the second set, and my player felt pressure, in what she thought should be an easy win. Why was it now, an even match in the second? She was visually and mentally distracted. Her brother was standing in perhaps the worst possible place, in the direct sun light, a few feet from the fence in line with the center line. I asked him to move to a spot in the shade, off to the side, so that he would not appear to be ever present.

**I also asked him not to get direct eye contact with his sister.**

On a changeover I asked her how she was doing, and she burst out into tears, saying that, 'all my problems have come back to me right now'. She had been making some bad errors, but now it was worse, and her good shots weren't struck very well. She needed less anxiety in her life. I asked her to simply think about playing well, breathing and seeing the ball coming out of the opponent's frame. She steadied herself, but a couple poorly timed errors meant she lost the second set and went into a third set match tiebreaker to 10. The last score I heard was 5-1 for the opponent, as I had other matches to watch. The tiebreaker went on and on, any moment, I expected to see her shake hands, lose, and burst into tears. It seems I missed every point she won, two out of the three points I saw, she lost, but finally my girl came out on top 12-10. She wasn't able to see the ball well, having a relaxed concentration when her mind was distracted. Once we were able to salvage some semblance of ball awareness, she was able to eke her way out of that match, with a victory. These kinds of successes can only happen if the visual skills are trained previously.

**These are also not the normal stories that are told in tennis books, but they are the types of things that commonly happen.**

# About the Author

Bill Patton is a Maverick Leader and has always colored outside the lines. He used to take his toys apart to see how they worked. He turned those experiences into a strength. Now he creates innovative templates so that others can build on success and make it their own. He is most proud of winning an NCS Championship, and becoming a published author for the first time. While his efforts on social media are to bring a convention a day experience, so you don't have to travel, he is also available to speak to your group. Bill travels to different parts of the country to talk with industry leaders, coaches workshops, and high school groups.

Bill is a Tennis Professional and is currently coaching his 8th different high school with 30+ years of experience in the field. He has coached at several schools with many great results. Mainly, the players had a great time maximizing their games, and playing on the teams. You can find videos, and podcasts featuring Bill, and he is easy to find on social media. He is married with two adult children. He is now a Senior Contributor with SportsEdTV.com, the most active sports instruction website in the world and was formerly certified at the professional level by the largest teaching organizations in the US: PTR and USPTA. Bill also has been heavily influenced the Evolutionary Sports Collective, with the caveat that he differs on some issues with the group. You can also catch some periodic articles in the Tennis Business Newsletter.

For more information, and/or about becoming Visual Training for Tennis Certified, email me at infinitevisioncoach@gmail.com. Visual Bill on Facebook, BillPatton720 on Instagram and many other minor platforms, Bill Patton on Clubhouse.

Printed in Great Britain
by Amazon